STRENGTH AND CONDITIONING FOR DANCERS

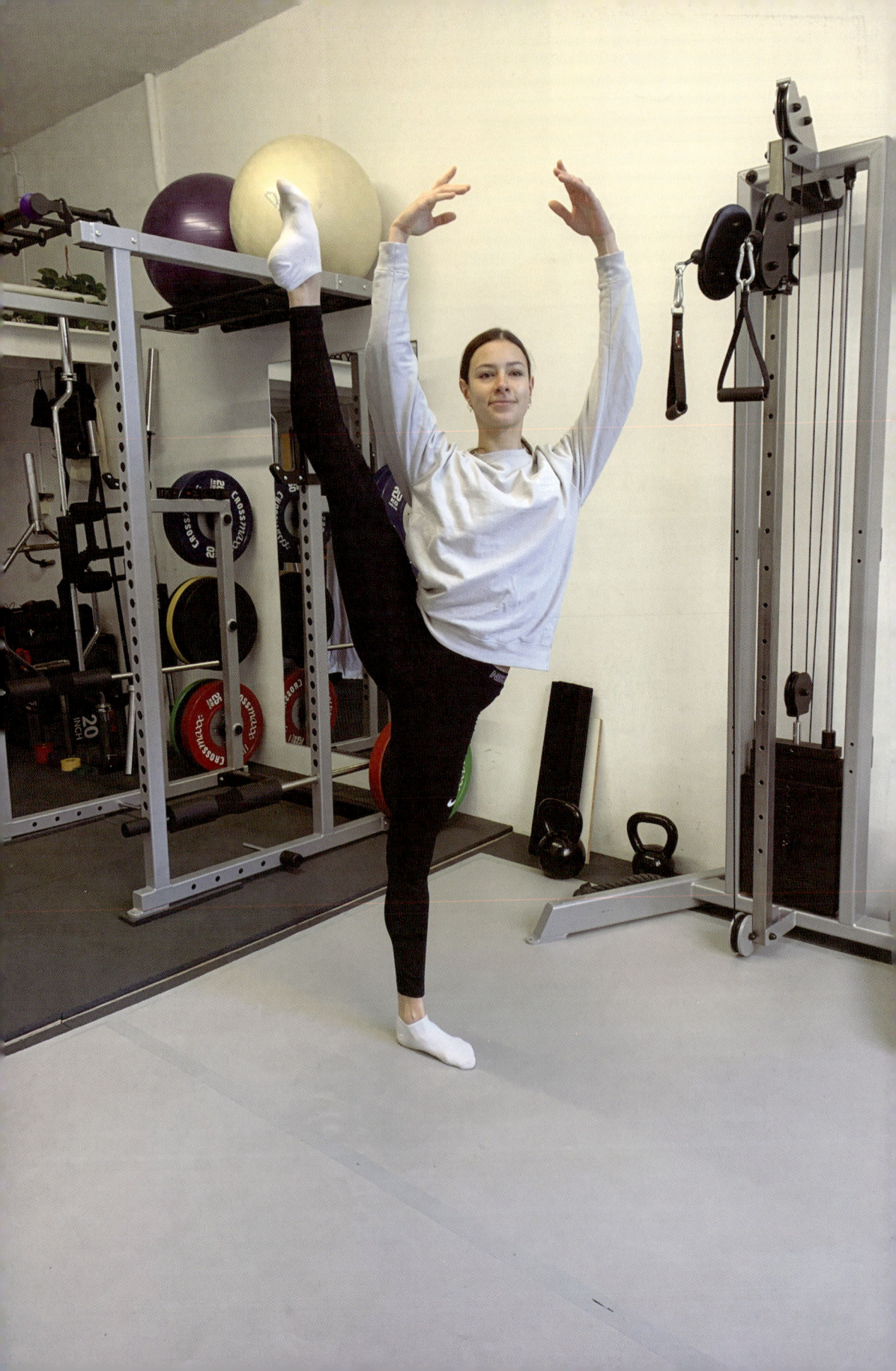

STRENGTH AND CONDITIONING FOR DANCERS

THE CROWOOD PRESS

First published in 2021 by
The Crowood Press Ltd
Ramsbury, Marlborough
Wiltshire SN8 2HR

enquiries@crowood.com
www.crowood.com

© Matthew Wyon and Sefton Clarke 2021

All rights reserved. No part of this publication may be reproduced or transmitted in any form or by any means, electronic or mechanical, including photocopy, recording, or any information storage and retrieval system, without permission in writing from the publishers.

British Library Cataloguing-in-Publication Data
A catalogue record for this book is available from the British Library.

ISBN 978 1 78500 977 8

Cover design: Blue Sunflower Creative

Typeset by Simon and Sons
Printed and bound in India by Parksons Graphics

CONTENTS

Acknowledgements 6

Preface 7

Introduction 10

1 THE FUNDAMENTALS..13
2 TRAINING PRINCIPLES..22
3 TRAINING THE DIFFERENT ATHLETIC COMPONENTS 31
4 SCREENING AND PROGRAMME DESIGN..................................47
5 PILATES FOR DANCERS – by Aline Nogueira Haas 67
6 CORE EXERCISES 76
7 LOWER-BODY EXERCISES 87
8 UPPER-BODY EXERCISES..121
9 PLYOMETRICS 138
10 PROGRAMME IDEAS TO GET YOU STARTED 150
11 DANCE NUTRITION – by Tommy Zarate 158

References 171

Index..174

ACKNOWLEDGEMENTS

Matthew and Sefton would like to thank Lore Zonderman and Joseph Massarelli (Dutch National Ballet), for giving up their time to be our photo models.

Matthew: I would like to thank my family for giving me the space to write. Also Jackie Pelly and Sharon Morrison, formerly the respective physiotherapists at English National Ballet and Birmingham Royal Ballet, for allowing me to provide pre-season and individual training for the dancers in their companies all those years ago. Paul Thacker, a friend and S&C collaborator, who helped me develop; and the dancers I have had the privilege to work with over the past 25 years.

Sefton: I would like to thank Simona and Sophie for their patience, understanding and generally putting up with me. Also Derrick Brown for mentoring me throughout my career, and Orlando Goacher for being there and guiding me.

Thanks to Dutch National Ballet and National Ballet Academy of Amsterdam for allowing me to begin my S&C path with them. And to all the dancers I have had the honour of dancing and working with, in and out of the gym over the years.

> There are two kinds of truth: the truth that lights the way, and the truth that warms the heart. The first is science, and the second is art. Neither is independent of the other or more important than the other. Without art, science would be as useless as a pair of high forceps in the hands of a plumber. Without science, art would become a crude mess of folklore and emotional quackery. The truth of art keeps science from becoming inhuman, and the truth of science keeps art from becoming ridiculous.
>
> *The Notebooks of Raymond Chandler*, Ecco Press, New York, 1938

PREFACE

ABOUT THE AUTHORS

Matthew Wyon

Matthew Wyon PhD, is a Professor in Dance Science at the University of Wolverhampton, UK. He is a founding partner of the National Institute of Dance Medicine and Science (NIDMS) UK, was the President of International Association for Dance Medicine & Science in 2015–17 and is the Chair of the IADMS Professional Development Committee. He started working as a strength and conditioning coach with ballet and contemporary (modern) dancers in the 1990s and this stimulated his thirty-year focus on how dancers can be supported to maximize their performance potential. Through NIDMS he continues to provide support, as an applied physiologist, to individual dancers and companies.

> When working with student and professional dancers in both contemporary/modern dance and ballet as an S&C coach I have found their technical ability surpasses their physical fitness abilities. Although the dancers were capable of carrying out amazing jumps and lifts, there was not the physical fitness back-up to prevent faulty technique creeping in as they became fatigued. I noted that the effects of fatigue started more rapidly than in other more conditioned athletes I was training. Also, the effect of always doing high-skill movements in their training and performances meant that few dancers were used to working at a high intensity (you have to decrease the intensity you work at as the skill element increases).[1] One of the main tasks was to build a solid foundation of physical fitness before gradually getting the dancers used to working at these higher intensities.
>
> Some important learning points, for myself, included the following:
>
> - their commitment to excellence is no different from any elite athlete; the performance goals are just different
> - there is often a focus on what they are good at rather than what they need to develop
> - you need to understand what they do and are currently doing, so watch class and rehearsals and talk to them about what they want to develop
> - although dancers can pick up new training exercises very quickly, you still need to progress slowly, so their underlying physiological structures develop adequately
> - they are not used to DOMS (localized muscle pain, covered in Chapter 2) so you need to develop their foundation fitness slowly
> - they are already doing a lot of exercise, so what seems to be a minimal amount of intervention has a beneficial effect
> - the aim is not to produce an Olympic power athlete, but an athletic artist who has an improved physical fitness reserve to support their artistry

Sefton Clarke

Sefton Clarke danced professionally at an elite level for almost twenty years in some of the most prestigious classical companies worldwide, The Royal Ballet, Birmingham Royal Ballet, Düsseldorf, Zurich, Vienna and Dutch National Ballet where he was a soloist for twelve years. On retirement he went into the field of nutrition, health and strength and conditioning, travelling the world to learn the most up-to-date methodologies within these fields. With this experience and knowledge, he became the Strength and Conditioning coach for the National Ballet Academy in Amsterdam and the Dutch National Ballet. He gives seminars on training to doctors, physiotherapists, medical students and trainers, as well as lectures on nutrition to many of the top artistic schools in The Netherlands. He co-founded and wrote a fully accredited personal trainers' course that is now known throughout The Netherlands and accredited throughout Europe. Most recently he has opened up his own private studio where he gives training to professional dancers, actors and everyone in between.

> During a rehearsal I broke one of my toes landing from a jump. This was due to fatigue and loss of technique, two main factors that can cause injury. This was a turning point for me and where I began to ask questions about my own physical abilities and how I could improve them.
>
> At that time, S&C for classical dance was in its infancy and there was not a lot of research around, so I turned to the athletic world to learn and bring across aspects that I thought were useful and apply them to myself. This worked and I began to delve deeper into this area as the results were excellent: more strength, increased work capacity and greater recoverability.
>
> I continued with strength training and incorporated it into my schedule, making sure that I focused on addressing certain weaker areas that do not normally get trained during ballet class or rehearsals. As I gained strength this was not to the detriment of my dancing and only enhanced it. I was underweight to begin with, due to poor nutrition and lack of what I call 'cross-training'; this extra strength served not only to help protect but as an added bonus it helped with my aesthetics, making for better symmetry between my upper and lower body as well as creating better lines throughout.
>
> By this time, I had been strength training for a couple of years and due to the results other dancers had become interested in additional training outside of the ballet studio. I had gained a better understanding of how to programme workouts and what was needed, but there was still a reluctance to accept this sort of training for fear of 'getting bigger' – in part due to the stigma attached to weight training, even with the results staring the dancers in the face. I began to try and break down these myths and barriers by proving that it is possible to get stronger without necessarily getting bigger, because in the end 'strength is a skill' much like ballet is. It is something that requires patience and consistency, and with the right programming it will only help with a dancer's career without them becoming a bodybuilder. The outcomes between the two are entirely different and require different training methodologies.
>
> I began working with the medical team of the company to devise a way of incorporating strength training into the dancers' already overburdened schedule. One of the ways we did this was by breaking a programme down into components that were manageable and would allow the dancer to complete a workout without overstressing their system. Over time this was refined and retuned with great results and the dancers were performing better than ever. This was further evidence that S&C can fit into the dance world in a way to suit everyone's needs.

Aline Nogueira Haas (Chapter 5, Pilates for Dancers)

Aline Nogueira Haas started her studies in Pilates with Romana Kryzanowska in 1998, and she was certified by 'The Pilates Studio' in 1999. In 2006, she finished the 'Power

Pilates® Certification Program' and, in 2008, opened the second Power Pilates® Affiliate Studio in Porto Alegre, Brazil – ATC Power Pilates® South Region Brazil. She became a PMA Certified Teacher in 2010. She has been working with Pilates for more than twenty years in different ways: as an instructor, as a teacher trainer, and as a researcher. As an Associate Professor and Senior Researcher at the Federal University of Rio Grande do Sul, she has been researching and publishing papers on Pilates since 2014.

Tommy Zarate
(Chapter 11, Dance Nutrition)

Tommy Zarate is a Brazilian jiu-jitsu competitor and performance nutritionist supporting teams within the EFL and ECB. He is CISSN and SENr certified with an MSc in Sports Nutrition. Before relocating to the United Kingdom, Tommy set up his consultancy, The Performance Nutritionist, LLC, supporting various athletes from the United States, New Zealand, and Singapore. Previously, Tommy was enlisted as a combat medic in the United States Army where he fought in OEF IX during the Global War on Terrorism. His hobbies include international travel, street photography, and eating.

There are two kinds of truth: the truth that lights the way, and the truth that warms the heart. The first is science, and the second is art. Neither is independent of the other or more important than the other. Without art, science would be as useless as a pair of high forceps in the hands of a plumber. Without science, art would become a crude mess of folklore and emotional quackery. The truth of art keeps science from becoming inhuman, and the truth of science keeps art from becoming ridiculous.

The Notebooks of Raymond Chandler, Ecco Press, New York, 1938

INTRODUCTION

What is Strength and Conditioning Training?

Strength and conditioning (S&C) training covers a wide range of activities that have the underlying aim to cause change to the body. Our body is a reactive organism that responds to increased or decreased levels of physical stress placed on it by adapting accordingly. Basically, by putting a regular new stress on the body it starts to adapt positively so that it can cope with this new stress easily; in the same vein, if we remove a stress from the body it starts to degenerate. In this context, the stress is focused on neuromuscular or cardiorespiratory systems of the body and activities can include Pilates, weight training, running and stretching. The stress can be generated by numerous means including bodyweight, bands, machines, weights, etc. It is how these stresses are placed on the body, the genetics and sex of the person, their training history, their nutrition – to mention a few factors – that will determine how the body reacts.

Depending on the training status of an individual, training adaptations can occur both centrally and peripherally. Generally, central adaptations occur prior to peripheral ones and can include refining or developing motor skills, development of the central cardiorespiratory system (heart and lungs), and enhancement of the biofeedback mechanisms. Peripheral adaptations include the development of supply mechanisms (increasing capillary bed density in the muscles and glycogen content of the muscle cells), increase in specific enzyme concentrations in the muscle cells involved with particular energy (ATP) replacement systems, and the structural adaptation of muscle fibres and tendons.

Supplemental S&C training has become a regular aspect of training for sportspeople involved with activities ranging from golf to powerlifting. It is incorporated to supplement skills training, to enhance performance or help protect the body against the forces it experiences that could lead to injury.

Dance too has been utilizing supplemental S&C training since the 1920s in the form of Pilates when Joseph Pilates opened his studio in the same building as the New York City Ballet. It was reported that his exercises allowed them to dance better and promoted the aesthetic that Balanchine and other choreographers came to favour: long lean limbs with large ranges of movement that needed to be supported by a strong core. In the 1950s, Audrey de Vos started to incorporate anatomical knowledge and conditioning exercises into the dance class to enhance performance. Other dance genres incorporated somatic techniques into their training as either a philosophical approach within a technique class or as supplemental training. For a long time, somatic training was the main supplemental training that dancers engaged in and it wasn't until the 1990s that other forms of training started to become more established.

In the 1990s, Professor Craig Sharp referred to dancers as 'artist athletes' due to the physical demands and training requirements of dance. Their long training days and performance demands were often in contrast to that seen in other sports, in which there had been a change from quantity to quality

INTRODUCTION

training and reduced performance/competition schedules (their epiphany moment had occurred twenty to thirty years earlier). The forty-hour training weeks with 200 plus performances a year that ballet dancers in the UK were contracted for was in sharp contrast to sport; soccer players, for example, were training around four hours a day and played approximately fifty matches a year. Dance, in nearly all its professional forms, has a culture of striving for perfection through long hours of training reinforced by the '10,000 hours to make a dancer' dogma.

EVIDENCE FOR WHY S&C SHOULD BE INCORPORATED INTO DANCE TRAINING

From the mid-twentieth century, medical professionals working with dance companies were noting a high incidence of injuries and suggested the need for healthcare screening, physical fitness training and special classes for injured dancers returning to dance.[2] Subsequent research in the 1980s noted little change in conditions[3] and led to the Fit to Dance[4] research and surveys. This provided empirical and self-reported data that suggested dancers were not physically or mentally prepared for the demands of their profession.[5] Subsequent research has highlighted areas of physical conditioning that have been either linked to injury incidence or performance enhancement. Over a number of studies Koutedakis and colleagues indicated that there is a link between leg strength and injury incidence with weaker dancers being more prone to injury.[6] Other researchers noted that there was a mismatch in the stresses placed on the cardiorespiratory system during dance class and rehearsal and the ensuing performance.[7] These empirical studies were reinforced by self-reported data from surveys[4,8] that indicated dancers felt that the main causes of injury were being fatigued and overworked, a fact that Koutedakis showed when dancers became fitter with rest, an indication that they were overtrained.[9] It wasn't until the early 2000s that research started to provide evidence of the link between physical fitness and performance enhancement. Twitchett and colleagues (ballet)[10] and Angioi et al. (contemporary/modern dance)[11] showed that fitter dancers were perceived to dance better by external dance experts and the dancers were injured less.[12,13]

There can be considered to be three main training phases: dancers move from pre-vocational training to vocational or pre-professional training and finally become professional dancers. Each of these phases has a different focus and goals, though there are elements that will flow through all three. 'Training age' is an important term; it refers to the number of years you have been training for a particular activity. It refers to the accumulated work and skill built up over a period of time. A professional twenty-year-old dancer who has been training since they were five years old has a dance training age of fifteen years; but if they have only been doing supplemental fitness training since the age of eighteen, their strength and conditioning training age is just two years. An important observation we, the authors, have seen over the past twenty years training dancers is that dancers can learn the correct technique for different strength training moves very quickly. There is often a tendency to increase the resistance too quickly because of the good technique, but this can be detrimental, as the underlying physical structures (muscles, tendons, ligaments) have not developed at the same rate and can leave the dancer vulnerable to injury. Dance is full of long-held beliefs that certain forms of exercise are 'taboo' for dancers, that they can cause muscular hypertrophy, develop the wrong muscles or wrong look/aesthetic, decrease flexibility, etc; often top of the list are weight training and running. As part of this book, we will discuss these myths and how supplemental

INTRODUCTION

training can be incorporated into schedules that will benefit the dancer.

Unfortunately, the dance world is still lacking in provision in this area and could benefit greatly from it. Over the decades the aesthetic in classical dance has changed and the demands are greater – more streamlined bodies, higher legs, bigger jumps, more extreme positions – but the strength and conditioning levels to be able to perform these have not adjusted accordingly, and herein lies the problem.

In this day and age, S&C training should not just be supplemental training in a dancer's life but an actual requirement programmed into the season, as this will not only reduce the risk of injury and help with overtraining, it will also, perhaps, help the dancers to have a longer and healthier career.

1 THE FUNDAMENTALS

Introduction

We are designed to move in a bipedal fashion and our body's structure has developed to optimize this type of movement with its skeletal structure and muscle organization. But within this uniformity of being human, there is a lot of individual variation that can affect how we move. This chapter looks at the basics of how we move and control movement.

Body Composition

Body composition is often viewed as a controversial topic within dance and this section aims to remove some of the 'politics' associated with it and focus on some of the important issues. Individual differences are due to our stature, frame size, age, activity levels, genetics and nutritional practices. Our weight can be 'divided' up into a number of different categories that can include muscle weight, bone weight and fat weight (this can be sub-divided into storage and essential fat).

At a basic level, Body Mass Index (BMI) has often been used for the general adult population to indicate health.[14] This is calculated by dividing body mass (weight in kg) by height (metres squared) and provides a score that if between 20–25 is considered healthy and above 30 to be obese with increased health issues. At the other end of the scale, scores below 18 have been linked to ill-health as well (amenorrhea for females and osteoporosis). For children and adolescents there are growth charts to use for comparison but again these are designed for the general population. BMI is a crude measure as it doesn't look at what the body weight is comprised of and often, muscle mass accounts for most of our weight and, depending on the activity a person is involved in, can lead to large variations in weight; elite athletes can be classified as clinically obese due to large amounts of muscle (rugby players) or underweight with comparatively little muscle mass (distance runners).

Our skeleton can account for 12–15 per cent of our total body weight. The variation is often due to the load it has to support with both increased muscle mass and fat mass requiring increased density and therefore weight. Skeletal growth is usually finished by eighteen to twenty years old, though minor accumulations in bone mineral density can still occur until thirty years old.[15] The bone density can also vary throughout the body: generally our lower body has greater bone mineral density than our upper body as it has to cope with

THE FUNDAMENTALS

	Males	**Females**
Height	172 cm	165 cm
Weight	70 kg	56.8 kg
Muscle	31.4 kg (44.8%)	20.5 kg (36%)
Bone	10.5 kg (15%)	6.8 kg (12%)
Total fat	10.5 kg (15%)	15.4 kg (27%)
Storage fat	8.4 kg (12%)	8.5 kg (15%)
Essential fat	2.1 kg (3%)	6.8 kg (12%)

Table 1 Example body composition comparison for the sexes.

the impact of moving and these areas are protected to the detriment of less stressed areas. This is certainly an issue for dancers; numerous studies have reported that dancers have similar or greater bone mineral density (BMD) in their femur, pelvis and lower back than the general population but much lower densities in the upper body with a greater fracture risk.[16] Interestingly, increasing stress through these regions through supplemental fitness training can increase the BMD.

Both males and females have essential fat, encompassing protective fat around organs (the heart, liver, spleen, kidneys, intestine, muscles and reproductive organs), the fat in bone marrow and throughout the central nervous system; females have a higher percentage than males, mainly to do with the protection of the uterus and ovaries and breast content. Storage fat comprises the rest of our body's fat component and again a certain amount is essential for our health and daily living but in the general sedentary population, it is the amount of storage fat that people carry that has negative health implications. Very low body fat levels can have major ill-health effects for both males and females; for both sexes there is an increased risk of asthma,[17] 'run-down' illnesses such as coughs and colds,[18] and also increased risk of injury and time it takes to recover from an injury.[19] For females the implications are heightened, with low body fat leading to amenorrhoea[20] (irregular or total loss of menstruation) and increased risk of osteoporosis.[20,21]

MUSCLES

Muscles have four behavioural properties: extensibility, elasticity, irritability and tension. The first two refer to a muscle's ability to be stretched or increase in length (extensibility) and the ability to return to its normal length after being stretched (elasticity). A muscle's elasticity also helps with the smooth transmission of tension from the muscle to the bone. A muscle has two types of elastic component: parallel (PEC) and series (SEC). PEC is provided by the muscle membranes (endomysium, perimysium and epimysium) and provides the resistance when a muscle is passively stretched. The SEC is from the tendons and as we will examine later can act as a spring, storing elastic energy during the stretch-shortening cycle of locomotion. Both SEC and PEC are primarily made up of collagen which has a viscous property that allows stretch and recoil but can also be lengthened over time if the correct stimulus is applied to it. Collagen is found throughout the body and its properties change over time; when we are young it has a wavy formation with few cross bridges between fibres (this is what allows it to stretch) but as we get older the wavy formation lessens and more cross

THE FUNDAMENTALS

bridges appear, thereby reducing its extensibility. This ageing effect can be mitigated by continued activity that promotes stretching muscles.

The irritability and tension properties of muscles correspond to their ability to respond to a stimulus. These can be either mechanical or electrochemical. The former refers to how a muscle responds to an external blow by contracting to prevent potential damage if it is stretched. The electrochemical stimulus denotes the action potential from nerve stimulation.

Muscle anatomy

A muscle's gross anatomy comprises of muscle fibres covered in endomysium (connective tissue that also contains capillaries and nerves) bundled together with perimysium (more connective tissue) to make a fascicle; these in turn are bundled together and encased by epimysium, a fibrous connective tissue, to make a muscle. All these connective tissues (endomysium, perimysium and epimysium) are continuous with each other and the tendon and make up what is often referred to as the fascia.

At a micro-level, muscle fibres are made up of bundles of myofibrils and this is where muscle contraction actually occurs. Along the length of a myofibril there are a series of Z-lines (named because of their shape) and attached to these are actin filaments (I-band). Between the Z-lines are M-bands made up of myosin filaments; where the actin and myosin filaments overlap is referred to as the A-band. As the actin and myosin slide together the A-band gets bigger and the I and M bands get less, and the length of the myofibril shortens. When this is extrapolated across thousands of myofibrils, across thousands of muscle fibres and fascicles a muscle shortens or contracts. As the actin and myosin 'slide' together by forming, releasing and reforming a series of cross-bridges the A-band increases and it is this, the number of cross-bridges between the actin and myosin filaments, that determines the force or tension a muscle generates.

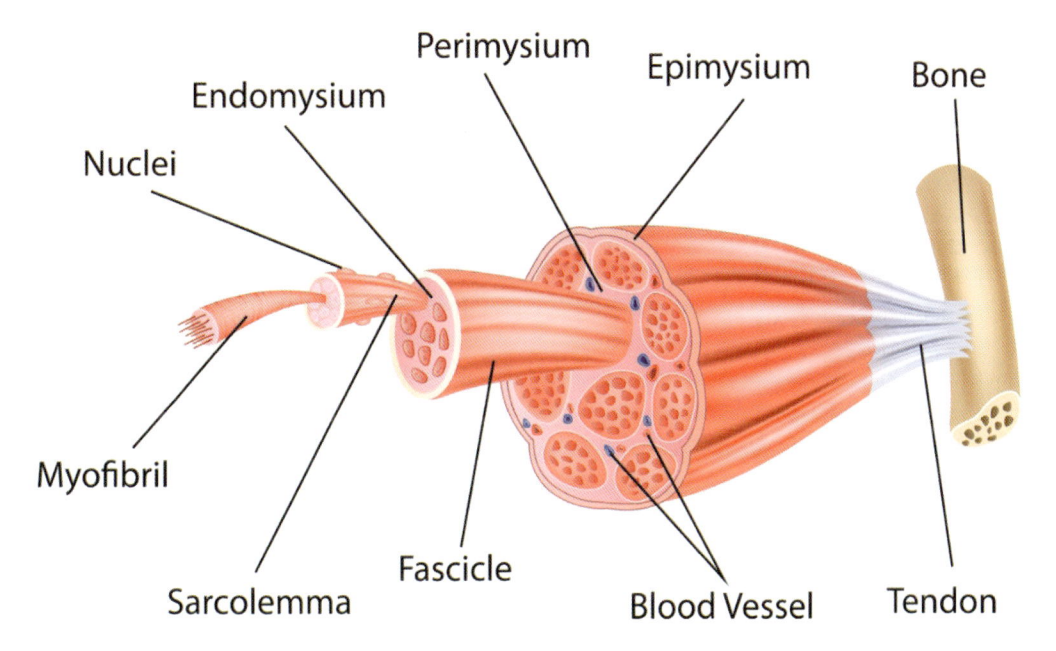

Fig. 1 Anatomy of a muscle.

Muscle fibres

There are a number of ways of categorizing muscle fibres; at its most basic, muscle fibres are either fast or slow twitch. This relates to the speed at which they contract, fast twitch (FT) approximate $100 m.s^{-1}$ and slow twitch (ST) $50 m.s^{-1}$, which in turn is determined by how quickly energy is made available for the cross-bridge cycling. The composition of FT and ST fibres in a muscle is predominantly determined genetically by the DNA given to you by your parents and can't be changed.[22] Fibres can be further categorized according to a variety of characteristics (Table 2).

As can be seen from Table 2, FT-A fibres can take on some of the characteristics of ST fibres and these adaptations occur due to the training stresses they are exposed to.[23]

Fibre architecture

Fibre architecture refers to how muscle fibres are organized in relation to the tendon. Different arrangements influence muscle function including the amount of force it can generate and the amount it can stretch (range of movement). There are two main arrangements: parallel, where fibres are orientated in parallel with the longitudinal axis of the muscle and can include sphincter/circular muscles; and pennate, where the fibres lie at an angle to the longitudinal axis. Parallel arrangements have more extensibility potential but can generate less force than pennate arrangements (an example is the bicep). Muscles that are required to generate a lot of force mostly have a pennate arrangement. This is because more fibres can be packed in, thereby generating more force. The angle of attachment is important: if it is greater than 60 degrees then only around 50 per cent of fibre force is transmitted to the tendon. There are a number of pennate arrangements: unipennate, where fibres are arranged solely on one side of the tendon (e.g. extensor digitorum); bipennate, where fibres are arranged on both sides of the tendon (e.g. rectus femoris); multipennate, multiple pennate muscle configurations (e.g. deltoid). The pectoralis major has a slightly different fibre arrangement than is covered by pennate or parallel; it is known as 'convergent' as the fibres are in a fan arrangement converging onto a single tendon attachment.

Fibre Type	Slow Twitch (ST)	Fast Twitch A (FT-A)	Fast Twitch B (FT-B)
Contraction time	Slow	Fast	Very fast
Size of motor neuron	Small	Large	Very large
Resistance to fatigue	High	Intermediate	Low
Activity used for	Aerobic	Long-term anaerobic	Short-term anaerobic
Force Production	Low	High	Very high
Mitochondrial density	High	High	Low
Capillary density	High	Intermediate	Low
Oxidative capacity	High	High	Low
Glycolytic capacity	Low	High	High
Major storage fuel	Triglycerides	Glycogen, Creatine phosphate	Glycogen, Creatine phosphate

Table 2 Characteristics of the three main muscle fibre types.

THE FUNDAMENTALS

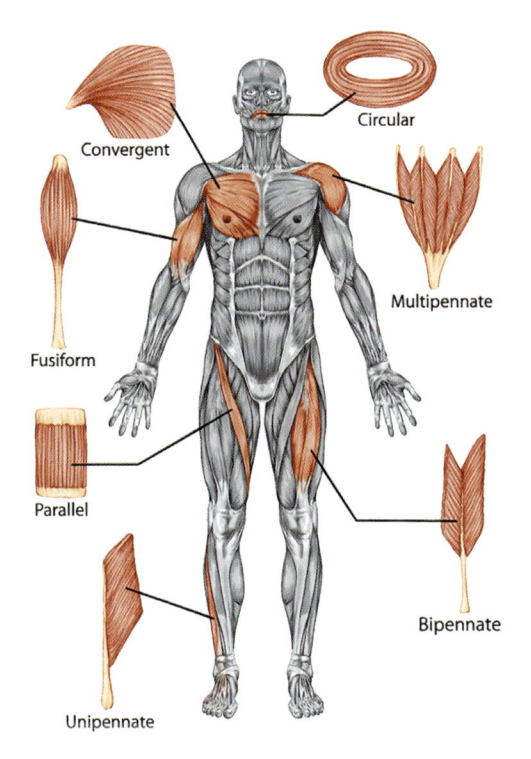

Fig. 2 The architecture of different muscles (with permission from PE.com).

MOVEMENT CONTROL

In its most basic form, movement is achieved by signals being sent from the brain causing specific muscles to contract; this reduction in muscle length causes bones to move around joint axes and movement is achieved. This is an extremely simplified description of a very complex task that is referred to as motor learning (ML) and although this is not the focus of this book it is important to understand some of the basics. From birth we start to learn to co-ordinate movement and as we get older our movements become more refined and accurate.[24] Within dance this is taken to an extreme, but the underlying principles are the same.

Our brain, referred to as the Executive in ML language, receives input from our surroundings, previous movements, etc., to determine what it needs to do next; this is the Response Period. It then chooses a 'motor programme' to carry out a specific task based on this evidence and sends signals to the appropriate muscles to cause a movement, the Effector Phase. During the movement, minute adjustments are made through feedback mechanisms such as muscle reflexes and ambient vision. All the while the brain is receiving Proprioceptive and Exteroceptive feedback on what the movement 'looked' like. Proprioceptive feedback refers to the internal feedback systems we have, including muscle spindles (information on how long each muscle is), Golgi tendon organs (feedback on the amount of force a muscle is exerting), cutaneous receptors (measuring pressure, temperature and touch), joint receptors (measuring forces within the joint), the vestibular system (detecting movements of the head and its relationship to gravity). Exteroceptive feedback is the information we receive from outside of the body. The main one is vision and we use both the focal (what it is) and ambient feedback to provide information on our environment (spatial and temporal aspects of our own movement, anticipation of upcoming events, movement of objects/people). Our auditory senses deliver information such as sound, movement of other dancers and verbal feedback from others.

We use all this information to compare what we thought the movement should look like, with what it actually looked like. This information is then used to adjust the motor programme to reduce the error within the movement. One of the issues when we start to learn new movements, is we receive enormous amounts of feedback and an important aspect of learning is deciding on what feedback mechanisms we should 'listen to', to help perfect the movement as quickly as possible. Skilled performers and learners have the ability to receive and process this vast amount of information quickly and accurately and to make effective adjustments when

THE FUNDAMENTALS

needed as they have learned what feedback to filter out.[25]

Another aspect of motor learning is found at the junction of the nerve and the muscle, the motor end plate. When enough nerve signals reach the end plate, a chemical is released that travels the very short distance between the nerve and the muscle and causes a muscle contraction. This is known as the 'All or Nothing Law': unless the threshold of nerve signals is reached at the end plate there won't be a contraction. Training helps reduce the number of nerve signals required before a contraction takes place. Each motor end plate controls a number of muscle fibres; the ratio of motor end plate to muscle fibres relates to the task a muscle is generally used for. In muscles that are involved with locomotion and gross movements one motor end plate can control thousands of fibres, whilst those involved with precision movements can contain only a few fibres. Through practice the motor programme learns how many motor end plates need to be activated to generate the required amount of muscular force for the desired action. Another important aspect of the motor learning is the timing of contractions over numerous muscles that allows co-ordinated movement. Part of our evolutionary neuromuscular development are agonist–antagonist pairings; these are particularly focused on locomotion. Part of their neuromuscular control means that when one is contracting, the other is relaxed, as its ability to receive nerve signals is blocked.[26] The exception to the rule is when one of the muscles in the pairing acts across two joints. An example of this is the quadriceps–hamstring pairing: because the hamstring causes hip extension as well as knee flexion, during a plié both are contracting eccentrically (lengthening under tension) and concentrically (shortening under tension) on the way up.

Muscle roles within movement

Muscles can take on one of five roles within a movement scenario as determined by the motor programme. The prime force generator is called the *agonist* muscle and opposing this muscle's action is the *antagonist* muscle, which can control the resulting movement effect of the agonist muscle by acting as a brake (especially during fast movements); an example is the quadricep–hamstring pairing. *Assistant agonists* are muscles that are involved in the movement as a force generator but are secondary to the primary agonist (e.g. the brachioradialis to the biceps brachii). *Stabilizers* are muscles that stabilize a region to prevent force dissipation from the agonist's action, the rhomboids act as stabilizers for shoulder movements. Finally, there are *neutralizers*, these prevent unwanted actions from the agonist muscle, for instance if the bicep brachii is contracting it can produce both flexion and supination but if the latter is not required then the pronator teres acts as a neutralizer.

Types of contraction

The term 'contraction' could be a slight misrepresentation of what a muscle can do to generate or cope with force as it indicates a shortening/contracting of the muscle. Muscles can either shorten, lengthen or stay the same length when coping with a force. The former is referred to as a concentric contraction, the next, eccentric contraction and the latter, an isometric contraction. When a muscle lengthens under force it can cope with much more force than during other types of contraction as these movements are often 'braking' in nature.

PHYSICAL FITNESS COMPONENTS

Physical fitness comprises a series of components that everyone possesses but depending on the activity that you are involved in, their importance can vary enormously. Dance as a generic term covers a multitude of different dance genres, all with different physical requirements and then within a specific genre the chorographical requirements, and therefore the physical demands, can vary drastically. The section on Needs Analysis (Chapter 4) will help you decide what needs to be focused on as primary and support components.

Physical literacy

Physical literacy refers to a biopsychosocial model[27] that incorporates movement competencies, rules and strategies of movement, motivation and behavioural skills of movement, and personal and social attributes of movement. Within the context of this book, we will focus on movement competency. Early specialization increases specific movement competencies to the exclusion of activities[28] in the belief that it will increase the likelihood of success. There is growing evidence that this is detrimental for children and young adolescents leading to increased risk of burnout, drop out, and a decrease in motor skill acquisition. Increasing the diversity of movement competencies is becoming more significant as choreography crosses different dance genres. If a professional dancer, especially a classical ballet dancer, has been denied this diversity of movement then they will find it harder to cope with the movement patterns required for more contemporary choreography. Also, only doing specific movement patterns day-in, day-out increases the risk of overuse injuries, the most prevalent type in dance.[29] Therefore, there is a need to increase the physical literacy of every dancer irrespective of age by doing a diversity of movement activities; strength and conditioning is one of these.

Cardiorespiratory fitness

This is a measure of how well we can cope during, and recover from, exercise. It is mostly focused on our ability to provide oxygen to our muscle fibres so that they can replenish the energy that has been used. Although this is often split into three main energy replenishment pathways, one aerobic and two anaerobic pathways, at a cellular level all pathways are working all the time to a greater or lesser extent depending on how quickly energy has to be replaced. Dance has been classified as intermittent exercise, in that it moves between different intensities and rest periods, rather than continuous steady state exercise like marathon running.[7,30] This means that all the pathways need to be trained to a degree. Aerobic fitness or capacity is the foundation for intermittent exercise as it is not only important during the activity but also during recovery periods.[31] The more developed the aerobic capacity, the less the anaerobic pathways are engaged and also the faster the recovery. But if the aerobic system is developed too much, the ability to work at really high intensities is diminished as the anaerobic pathways haven't been developed, and this will impact the high-intensity elements of dance.

Muscle function

This encompasses muscle strength, power and endurance; but also provides joint and core stability and the functions mentioned above under Muscle Roles. How a muscle is trained has an effect on its ability to perform in a specific manner and often training plans are contrary to required outcomes.[32] There are slight crossovers between the different types of training, but it is minimal. Muscle strength refers to the amount of load or weight a muscle can move for 1 to 3 repetitions; the movements are often slow (although the intent of these movements is to move fast), so that both the fast and slow twitch fibres can be engaged to provide assistance. Muscle power denotes an ability to generate force quickly, as in jumping. Generally, the force development comes from the engagement of the fast twitch fibres and the force generated is less than that seen for strength training. It is often recommended that strength training occurs prior to power training

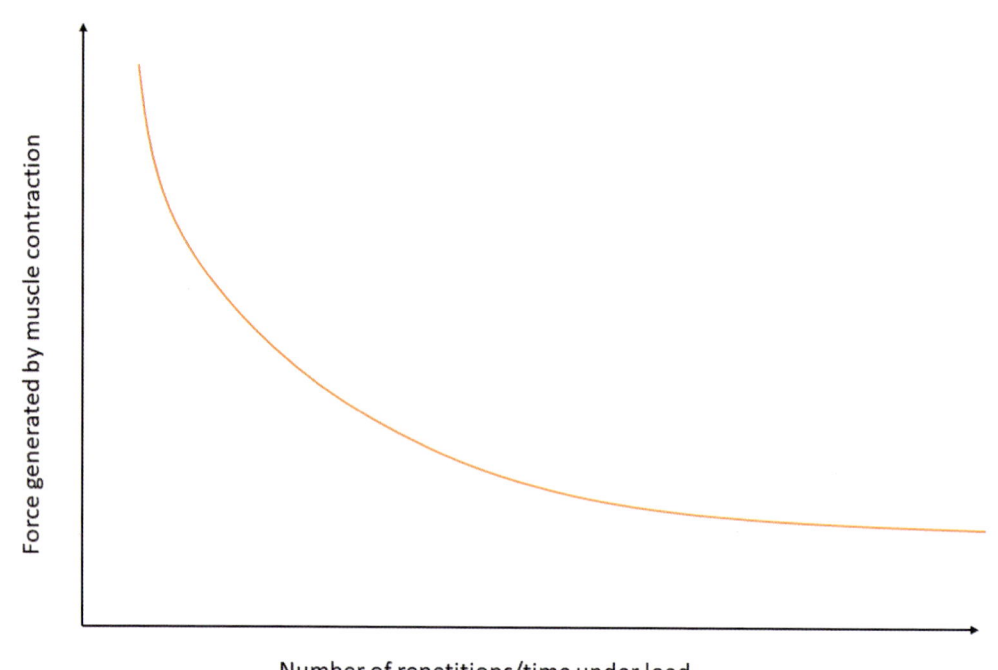

Fig. 3 The relationship between muscle force and number of repetitions.

as the former not only has a positive effect on the fast twitch fibres but it also strengthens the body's structures (tendons, ligaments, and stabilizer muscles) in preparation for power training. Muscle endurance refers to muscle contractions that occur over an extended period of time at a moderate to low force. In fact, the lower the force the longer the muscle can continue to contract.

An important aspect of muscle training is its neuromuscular component. In fact, the first stage of all muscle training sees development of this component. It refers to the improved co-ordination of the movement with the correct engagement and refinement of the primary agonists, assistant agonists and stabilizers. This will include learning to engage as many muscle fibres as possible at the same time for muscle strength, solely engaging the fast twitch fibres for muscle power and being about to rotate through a muscle's fibres for muscle endurance so that a fatigue effect is minimized.

Even though cardiorespiratory fitness and muscle training are often viewed as separate entities, how we train muscles will have a direct effect on the cardiorespiratory systems as muscle contractions use energy and the amount of force exerted, the number of repetitions carried out and the amount of rest between sets will challenge the cardiorespiratory replenishment systems. This is covered in more depth in the succeeding chapters.

Agility

This is the ability to decelerate, accelerate and change direction of movement without losing control of the body. It incorporates a lot of the other components of fitness such as muscle power, flexibility, balance and core stability so that a dancer can change direction quickly and effortlessly. Agility would seem to be inherent for nearly all dance genres, but it is a component that needs to be trained.

THE FUNDAMENTALS

Functional stability

This has often focused on the core, the lower torso between the pelvis and the ribs, but should encompass the whole body. How we control our limbs, both legs and arms, will affect how force or energy is transferred through the body. The lower torso is often focused on as this area has the least bony support, just the spine, and needs to be able to transfer forces generated by the legs or the arms to the rest of the body without folding or dissipating them. A functional whole-body approach, rather than an isolation method, has proven to have greater benefits.

Flexibility

This is the one component dancers are assumed to excel at, but it varies enormously between the genres. There is often a sex difference with females having greater range of movement (ROM), especially around the hips, than males. This is partly due to the skeletal structure of the pelvis that allows a greater ROM possibility but also female dancers' legs are generally slightly shorter and less muscular so there is less resistance. The resistance not only comes from the actual weight of the leg but also the internal resistance generated by the muscles being stretched, known as the parallel elastic component. Flexibility has a passive and active component; the former is how far a joint can be moved by an external force (another person or band) and the latter is how far we can move it using the agonist muscle to the one being stretched. Therefore, muscle strength is a component of flexibility (what is known as mobility). Ideally there should be little difference between passive and active ROM and also little bilateral differences (left and right); both have been shown to be an issue in some dance genres with greater ROM between the gesture leg and support leg and difference between active and passive ROM particularly in the gesture leg.

Balance and stability

Balance is your ability to control your equilibrium (centre of mass) when either static or moving at a constant speed, whilst stability is the ability to return to the balanced state after a disturbance to the equilibrium (change in direction, speed, movement) by moving the body. We are constantly moving between balance and stability states when dancing. These movements can be the minute adjustments made during a relevé or the arm and foot waving during a fouetté turn in an attempt to maintain balance. When it comes to training for stability, we have two reflexes within us: a righting reflex, which is moving and maintaining balance over a stable surface (such as dancing on stage or practising in the studio), and a tilting reflex, which is moving over an unstable surface (such as surfing or skiing).

Rest

Rest is one of the most important components of physical fitness and the one that often gets excluded or minimized. Rest allows your body to recover and repair itself, so the harder you train, the more planned rest you need. This mainly happens when you sleep and coincides with the importance of deep sleep when your repair hormones are released. Your body also needs longer periods of recovery on a weekly basis and if possible, you should have two rest or very light activity days a week, or at least one day as a minimum. On an annual basis it is also important to have time away from dancing and training; you can take up to 2 weeks away from all activity before the benefits of your previous training start to decrease. What has been noted is that at the end of the season dancers are often overtrained and require much longer periods of rest to recover.[9,33]

2 TRAINING PRINCIPLES

Our bodies are reactive mechanisms in that they adapt in response to a stimulus being added or taken away.[34] If a stimulus is new or greater than previously experienced then there is an anabolic (training) adaptation; if a stimulus is removed then there is a catabolic (detraining) adaptation. Interestingly, if a stimulus stays the same, the body learns to carry out the activity more efficiently and there is a slight detraining effect. Finding the appropriate stimulus can initially be a case of trial and error and involves your training age and physical competency.

Training Age

This refers to the number of years' experience you have in a particular activity. There can be some transference in training years between activities, but it depends on the similarities between the activities: the skills developed, primary muscles used, type of contraction, activity length, and force generated. Therefore, you could have a ballet training age of fifteen years, jazz training of five years, Pilates of five years and no years of strength training. One of the limitations of early specialization is that training years have been built up in one activity often to the exclusion of others, which can cause anatomical imbalances and also limit training age transference between different activities.

Physical Competence

This refers to an individual's ability to develop new movement skills and patterns. This is obviously highly developed within dancers and you, the dancer, can pick up new movements very quickly. The downside to this is that often the underlying anatomical development cannot develop at the same rate and this can leave you vulnerable to injury. Therefore, often a prolonged period of foundational training is required for the body's structures to develop sufficiently to keep up with your movement abilities.

Training Stimulus

The stimulus we place on the body needs to be specific to the goals we want to achieve, and these will be discussed in more detail in Chapter 4. For improvements to occur we need to stress a system beyond what it is used to. If too much stress is applied, then the system will break; if not enough, no improvements occur, or detraining can start to happen. This load can

TRAINING PRINCIPLES

be monitored in a number of different ways depending on the activities being undertaken.

Time under tension

This denotes the amount of time a muscle is under tension during a strength or power training session. It mainly refers to the work:rest ratio of a session – in other words, the number of repetitions of an exercise, the number of sets of repetitions, how long the muscle is under tension during the set, and the rest between the sets (for example, 4 sets of 10 repetitions with 2 minutes' rest between the sets). This, in combination with the force being exerted, will determine how a muscle adapts to the training stimulus. Increased time under tension (little rest between training sets) with high levels of force (training load) will have a hypertrophic effect (increases in muscle mass) as it has been shown to increase the release of testosterone, growth hormone and cortisol; a lower time (more rest between training sets) under tension with a similar training load will have a neuromuscular effect (increased co-ordination, fibre recruitment). The chosen training load also determines the time under tension: if a very heavy training load is chosen, the more rest is needed between sets to recover and therefore the adaptations become more neuromuscular; moderate to heavy training loads require less recovery, thereby increasing the time under tension and promoting hypertrophy; very light loads with lots of repetitions have long time periods under tension but because of the light load don't cause hypertrophy (the muscle may change shape but the volume rarely changes). Therefore, the amount of rest you have during a training session has a fundamental effect on how your muscle responds to training.

Weight moved

This refers to the total weight moved/lifted in a training session. For instance, a leg training session might encompass:

- Squats: 2 × 10 reps at 50kg; 2 × 6 reps at 100kg
- Straight leg deadlifts: 2 × 10 reps at 80kg; 2 × 6 reps at 100kg
- Calf raises: 4 × 15 reps at 80kg
- Therefore, the total weight moved for this session is 9,800kg

Training impulse (TRIMPS)

This is mainly used for cardiorespiratory training sessions. You record the length of the training session in minutes and multiply this by either the mean heart rate or rate of perceived exertion. Heart rate should be recorded/monitored via a chest band monitor to a watch, rather than solely via a watch, as the latter is less accurate. The Rate of Perceived Exertion, the sRPE ('s' refers to session), monitors how hard you felt the session was. This was developed by Borg,[35] who noted that perceived exertion was related to heart rate and developed a scale ranging from 6–20 (if you add a 0 to the numbers you get the equivalent heart rate to the perceived exertion); this has been further adapted to include a 1–10 scale as well. You can use either scale, though you need to be consistent in which one you choose. The top scores refer to maximal effort, whilst the bottom ones relate to resting states (Fig. 4).

Therefore a 20-minute session on a cross-trainer could be classified in the following ways:

Heart rate method	20 × 145 (mean heart rate during the session)	2,900
Borg Scale	20 × 15 (mean sRPE using 6–20 scale)	300
Modified Borg Scale	20 × 6 (mean sRPE using 1–10 scale)	120

Table 3 Recording sRPE.

Foot contacts

Quite simply this is the number of repetitions of high impact exercises that encompass hops,

23

TRAINING PRINCIPLES

Borg Scale	
6	
7	very, very light
8	
9	very light
10	
11	fairly light
12	
13	somewhat hard
14	
15	hard
16	
17	very hard
18	
19	very, very hard
20	

Modified Borg Scale	
0	at rest
1	very easy
2	somewhat easy
3	moderate
4	somewhat hard
5	hard
6	
7	very hard
8	
9	
10	very, very hard

Fig. 4 Rate of perceived exertion scales.

jumps and bounds. This monitoring system is usually solely used for plyometric training but can also be incorporated into dance training monitoring to record the number of jumps and hops in classes and rehearsals. This is particularly important after a holiday period when a gradual increase in contact loading has been shown to reduce the incidence of lower leg injuries such as shin splints.

Dance training

Your dance activities need to be taken into account as well, a number of studies have shown that sRPE is a valid measure of intensity across a number of dance genres.[36] Using the same model as TRIMPS, you multiply the sRPE by the length of the dance session (minutes) to calculate the session load.

MONITORING TRAINING LOAD

Generally, the body can cope with a 5–10 per cent increase in overall load a week; this is the accumulated load of all your activities – dance, supplemental training, rehabilitation, leisure activities – using the above training stimuli monitoring tools. Because you are training multiple components all at once it is imperative that it is the overall training load that increases each week, and not each component you are training. As dance is your primary activity (the other training components are there to support your dance), this training load takes precedence. Therefore, if your rehearsal and/or performance schedule starts to increase drastically then you might need to decrease the training load from supplemental training so

TRAINING PRINCIPLES

that the overall load remains within the 5–10 per cent band increase.

Each of the supplemental training components will have an individual importance for yourself depending on your current physical status and the demands of your dance schedule (see Needs Analysis in Chapter 4). As you can't train every component at the same time (see Scheduling Training section of this chapter) each component will have a descending level of importance, with some components being in 'maintenance mode' (trained just once a week to maintain previous improvements), whilst others are the main focus. When it comes to increasing your overall training load, it is the latter group that receives the increased training stimulus.

ADAPTATION AND SUPERCOMPENSATION

During exercise, muscles go through a catabolic period with the breakdown of molecules to release energy (ATP to ADP+Pi) and the breakdown/damage of muscle proteins. In the recovery or anabolic phase, the muscle cells work to replenish energy stores and repair the damaged protein structures (Fig. 5). If the training stimulus is more than previously experienced the muscle cells prepare to be able to cope with the new stimulus by either storing more energy or building more protein structures (hypertrophy), but if the training stimulus remains constant there is little or no adaptation (Fig. 5).

RECOVERY

Recovery is fundamental to optimal training, although it has taken a while to be recognized as an integral training component. Research has shown that depending on the type of training stimulus, the recovery time can vary quite markedly; this is measured in the time it takes for protein synthesis to return to normal levels post-exercise. As you can see from Fig. 6, intense anaerobic and strength training can take between 40 and 72 hours after the training session to recover; this doesn't mean you can't use those muscles in the interim period, but they won't be able to work optimally, and you are more likely to prolong the recovery period.

Nutrition also plays an important in the recovery process: if the right repair materials (mainly protein and carbohydrate) aren't available then it slows the process. Eating carbohy-

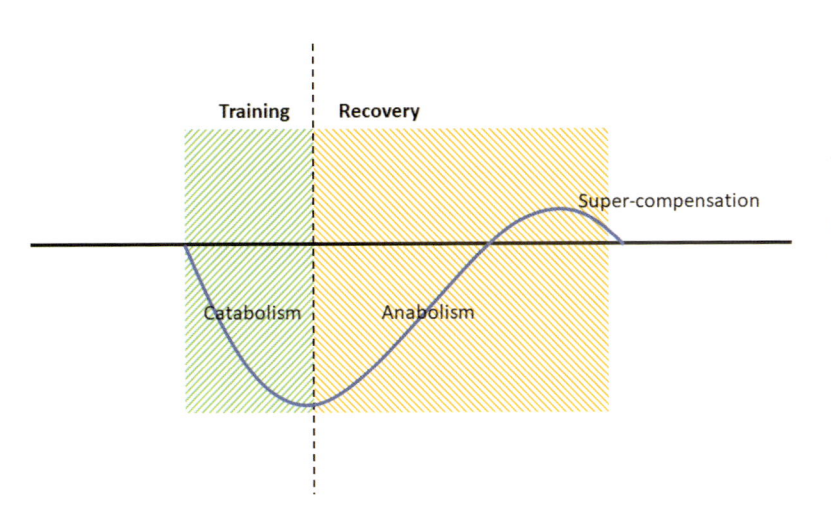

Fig. 5 The catabolic and anabolic effect of a single training session.

TRAINING PRINCIPLES

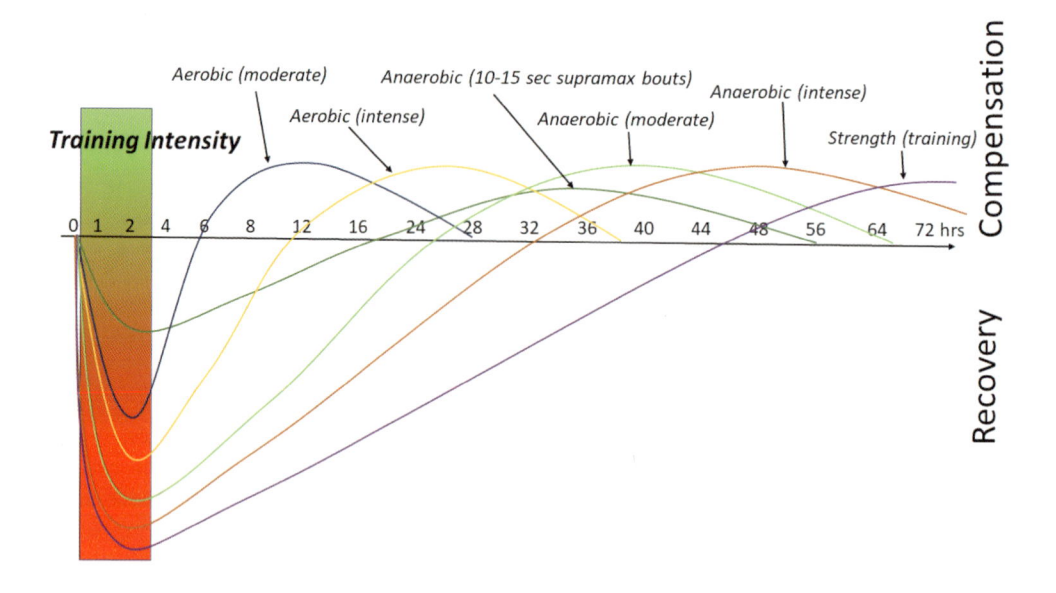

Fig. 6 Recovery periods for different training stimuli.

drate within 30 minutes of finishing a training session or performance has been shown to restore muscle glycogen (energy) stores faster, aiding the recovery process. In a similar manner, protein intake should be planned so that amino acids are available to coincide with the release of hormones associated with muscle repair (testosterone, growth hormone and insulin-like growth factors). A warm-down and low intensity stretching has also been shown to speed up recovery. The former helps with the removal of waste metabolites from the training session and the delivery of repair and replenishment molecules; the latter has been shown to promote healing better than higher-intensity stretching protocols.

Endocrine response

Post-exercise, the muscle fibre has increased levels of ADP and amino acids and these act as effectors for the protein synthesis. The main hormones involved with muscular repair and recovery are growth hormone (GH), insulin, insulin-like growth factors (IGF), and testosterone. They often work in conjunction; for instance, growth hormone also stimulates the release of IGF with the highest levels secreted at night. Growth hormone release is stimulated by muscle action and it increases amino acid (protein building blocks) transport into the muscle cell, protein synthesis within the cell, and also stimulates cartilage growth. IGF is a major stimulator of repair and building process in skeletal muscle. Its release is stimulated by training stress and GH, though IGF release has a 3–9 hour delayed response from initial GH release, again with peaks often occurring during sleep. Interestingly testosterone does not have as great an effect of muscle fibre recovery as IGF but it does promote GH release. Testosterone is also linked to the neuromuscular system by increasing the number of neurotransmitters and increasing the size of the neuromuscular junction, thereby increasing the number of fibres it controls. Both of these adaptations enhance a muscle's force production capabilities. Specific training modalities increase testosterone levels. These are heavy resistance exercises over multiple sets with short rest intervals; this response is seen in males rather than females.

Neuromuscular response

Initial increases in muscle strength are due to adaptive changes in the neuromuscular system, which optimize the muscle's response to the activity. The theoretical underpinning of the neuromuscular response and adaptation has been covered in Chapter 1. From an applied perspective this has a number of manifestations: to recruit the optimal number of muscle units and types of fibres for the task. Slow twitch fibres are recruited for muscular endurance activities, whilst fast twitch fibres are recruited for strength and power activities as well as eccentric muscle contractions; learning to engage the high threshold motor end plate units. These are only activated in maximal exertion situations, our fight or flight responses, but through training we can learn to recruit them for specific tasks. The neuromuscular system learns to 'rotate' through different fibre bundles in a muscle so that force production can be maintained over long periods of time, thereby delaying the onset of fatigue. The co-ordination of agonists, antagonists, assistant agonists, stabilizers and neutralizers for that movement pattern is improved and refined so the task can be completed with the minimum of effort and extraneous movement.

Delayed Onset Muscle Soreness (DOMS)

The localized muscle pain that can be felt one to two days after exercise is called DOMS. This is caused by microscopic tears in the muscle fibres, mainly from eccentric muscle movements. The body responds by increasing inflammation as this helps heal the damage but during this period the muscle is tender to touch, often has a reduced range of movement, there can be slight swelling of the muscle, and the muscle feels fatigued and weak. Every training session shouldn't cause DOMS, but it is normal to experience it when there is an increase in training intensity, eccentric training exercises or a new exercise is introduced.

Gentle exercise and stretching have been shown to help reduce the muscle soreness. Low- to moderate-intensity stretching,[37] cycling/swimming[38] and foam rolling[39] have been shown to help the recovery process; higher-intensity interventions are likely to exasperate the recovery process by increasing the muscle damage. Massage[40] and cryotherapy[41] as interventions have had mixed reviews on their physiological recovery benefits, though they might make you feel better.

Overreaching, supercompensation and overtraining

When you do excessive training, don't get enough recovery and start to experience excessive muscle soreness it starts to affect your ability to adapt and your physical performance abilities decline. In the short-term this is referred to as overreaching and recovery can be achieved with a few days' rest and sleep, proper nutrition, and reduced training volume and intensity. Sports coaches therefore often plan to put their athletes into an overreaching condition over a 6–8-week period before implementing a period of rest; this has been shown to result in significant increase in strength and power and is referred to as supercompensation. This would be difficult to implement within a professional dance company due to the performance demands, though it would be possible within a training institution.[42]

If a recovery plan isn't implemented, then there is a continued decline in physical performance, and this is referred to as overtraining or

TRAINING PRINCIPLES

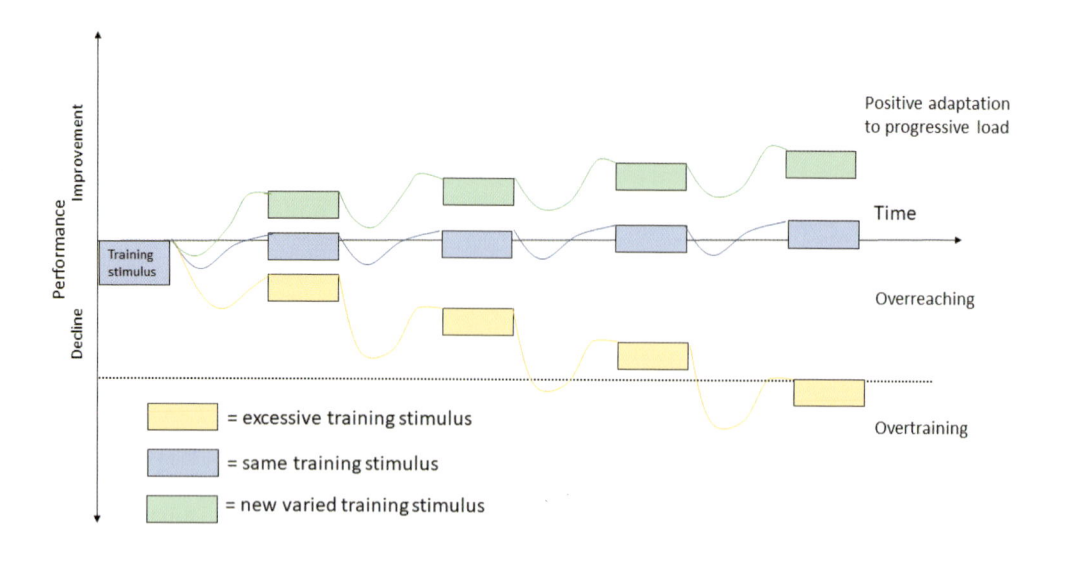

Fig. 7 The effect of optimal and sub-optimal recovery on long-term training.

burnout. This will require a more drastic period of rest and can last for a significant period of time. At the end of a performance session or academic year dancers are often close to this state and a period of rest (holiday) has been shown to actually improve physical fitness.[9]

Planning rest throughout the year is imperative, rather than relying solely on one long holiday; rest needs to occur on a daily, weekly and annual basis. Adequate sleep each day is required for our body's recovery (endocrine) systems to repair cellular damage caused by exercise and daily living. It is recommended that you should have at least one whole day off a week, or more if possible, to allow recovery and compensation to occur. If an extra half day can also be scheduled mid-week this would also help the process. Rest days need to be exactly that, and not an opportunity to do more or different exercise; very low intensity exercise such as Pilates or swimming for an hour is fine. Periods of reduced training intensity every 6–8 weeks is again recommended, though difficult to schedule within a dance environment. You need to consider rest a vital component of training as important as dance class and dance performance.

SCHEDULING TRAINING

Planning training sessions

Because dance schedules often change week by week within a professional dance or training school environment, we promote a series of 20–30-minute focused training sessions that can adapt to these schedules. This flexibility will allow you to decide how best to fit the supplemental training sessions into your schedule. There are some basic dos and don'ts that need to be followed so that the supplemental training does not have a negative effect on class, rehearsal, and performance schedules.

- Supplemental training can be both physically and mentally tiring, so plan your sessions carefully.
- Don't do weight training immediately before dancing, so try to schedule it at the end of the dance day. Weight training

causes short-term neuromuscular fatigue and therefore you won't be able to do high-skill or controlled movements in the 2–3 hours after a session.
- Train legs when you know you have a rest day the next day. The neuromuscular fatigue and muscle soreness can last 24–48 hours and as the majority of dance genres require a lot of leg work, a full recovery needs to be planned.
- Training for strength and power requires a lot of mental effort and focus, so don't try to train when tired and distracted.
- Cardiorespiratory training doesn't require much mental effort (with the exception of lactate training, see Chapter 3) and can be done at the end of the dance day.
- If you're tired, don't train. It is better to miss, or reschedule, a session rather than train tired, as you are more likely to get injured through poor technique or overloading a muscle beyond its current capacity.
- Quality is more important than quantity. Do your session and leave, rather than allowing it to become a social setting.
- Rest is training.

Training order

Cardiorespiratory and muscle function training

The health and fitness industry has nearly always promoted cardiorespiratory training before weight training; the thinking behind this is that the former will warm up the body for the latter and that if it is done the other way around, most people would skip, or shorten, the cardiorespiratory training. Also, for the general population, cardiorespiratory training has greater health benefits than weight training. Research suggests, however, that there is little difference between doing cardiorespiratory training before weight training or the other way around, as long as the person is motivated. The order should be determined by your goals: if your focus is cardiorespiratory development then this would take precedence over other interventions; if it is power then your main effort is focused here.

Training phases

Before 'dance specific' supplemental training can start, you need to prepare your body. The first phase is foundation training. This prepares the body for the next stage by focusing on muscle imbalances, stabilizers, synergists, and technique (not dance!). A screen from a physiotherapist is often a good idea at this stage to provide specialist input. All activity, if carried out for a long period of time, causes muscular imbalances; these can be either agonist–antagonist or bilateral (left–right). This only becomes an issue when the imbalance becomes greater than 10 per cent, as this has been shown to increase injury risk.[43] Stabilizer and synergist muscles are often relatively small but are vital during major movements. Their size means they can become a weak link within a movement, especially high force movements such as jumping, squatting and overhead lifting, leading to loss of alignment. The technique aspect is perfecting the movement patterns in the subsequent periods, whether this is weight training or cardiorespiratory training. If you start your training in the off-season, then another aspect of this period is to gradually increase the volume of your training; this needs to be in conjunction with, and respectful of, your dance training schedule.

The next phase focuses on the development of muscle strength and aerobic capacity; these form the real base for advanced training. Strength training is not only about increasing the amount of weight a muscle can move but also about strengthening the associated anatomical structures: tendon strength/thickness, joint ligaments, bone density, as well as improving inter-muscle co-ordination. Some of these adaptations are the accumulation of many years' training, particularly tendon and bone strength. Improving your aerobic capacity has both central and peripheral adaptations. The main central adaptation is the enlargement of the heart, especially the ventricles, allowing more blood and therefore oxygen to be pushed around the body per beat. Peripheral adaptations include increased capillarization of the muscles themselves, and in the fibres, increased mitochondria (a cellular structure where the main part of aerobic glycolysis occurs) and enzymes associated with glycolysis, increased myoglobin (similar to haemoglobin but actually in the muscle cell) and glycogen (stored glucose). You must remember that dancers aren't strength or endurance athletes but need these components as a base for more dance specific training. In both instances, improved strength and aerobic capacity allows all activities to be carried out at a lower percentage of your maximum capacity. Developing either of these components too much can have a detrimental effect on your dancing; both components result in 'slower' movement speeds than required for dance, hence they form the groundwork for the next two components.

The last phase encompasses power and anaerobic/lactate training. Both are often referred to as supramaximal training and require a lot of focused motivation to achieve the most benefits. These components 'turn' the benefits gained from the previous components into dance-specific adaptations. Power and plyometric training (Chapter 3) are about maximizing the amount of force that can be generated very quickly and focus on engaging the fast twitch fibres and reducing the 'amortization period' (the time between an eccentric and concentric contraction or between landing and taking off). This type of training requires the body to cope with high forces being rapidly applied to its structures and therefore power training needs to occur in a non-fatigued state so good alignment and quality of movement are maintained throughout. Power training focuses on neuromuscular adaptation particularly regarding the stretch–shorten cycle. For example, the calf muscle is stretched on landing from a jump and then contracts during take-off. As the calf muscle is acting as a break during landing, it is contracting eccentrically and the series elastic component (SEC, see Chapter 1) is stretched generating kinetic energy; if the amortization period can be reduced (the time at the bottom of a plié) then this stored kinetic energy can be added to the muscle's contractile forces thereby increasing the total amount of force generated, and resulting in a bigger jump. Anaerobic/lactate training is often referred to as High Intensity Intermittent Training (HIIT), though the HIIT training often espoused by the health and fitness industry has lost its physiological underpinnings and is just another name for circuit training. HIIT is interval training with particular work to rest ratios challenging specific energy replenishment pathways (Chapter 3), in this instance the lactate system. The importance of having a good aerobic base prior to HIIT training is that more high-intensity bouts can be achieved before fatigue occurs; the aerobic base helps increase the recovery between the bouts. The training is very tough as having high amounts of lactate in your system and muscles isn't at all pleasant and high levels of motivation are required to complete a training session.

The length of time spent within each phase is dependent on the time available and your current training status. As your dance training load increases with rehearsals, the amount of supplemental training should decrease, entering a maintenance phase. This refers to a minimal training stimulus that is enough to maintain your previous gains; this is particularly important during long performance periods or tours. Depending on the physical demands of rehearsals and/or performances, these could provide enough stimulus to maintain cardiorespiratory adaptations; strength and power components would probably need to be trained once a week.

3 TRAINING THE DIFFERENT ATHLETIC COMPONENTS

This chapter will provide detail on how to develop each athletic component and, where information is available, provide 'norms' for dancers. There is very little in the way of data on the latter and what is available doesn't necessarily relate to optimal capabilities. A lot of the published data will relate to reduced injury risk as there has been little research on optimal athletic development in relation to dance performance enhancement. S&C should be incorporated to support your dancing endeavours and currently there isn't the evidence that, for instance, increasing the amount you can squat from 1.5 times your bodyweight (BW) to 2 × BW has such an impact on your dance performance to justify the time taken to make that improvement in strength. The evidence mentioned in the introduction indicates that supplemental fitness training does have a beneficial effect on dance performance and injury incidence, and it should be part of a dancer's training to support and enhance their dance technique and performance virtuosity. The reasons for training each athletic component, how to train, and the benefits of each component will be outlined in this chapter, whilst the next chapter will provide you with ideas on how to develop appropriate training schedules based on your needs and screening; at its most basic, all regimens should be based on specificity ('how does this help me dance?') and overload[44] (progressive increase in training load).

CARDIORESPIRATORY TRAINING

Cardiorespiratory training is focused on developing the energy production pathways that replenish energy (ATP) levels in muscle cells. Muscle contraction uses up a muscle cell's ATP store at varying rates depending on the rate of cross-bridge cycling and then 'chooses' the most appropriate pathways to try to maintain the cell's ATP concentration. Your muscles will never run out of ATP as self-protective mechanisms step in to reduce the rate of contraction, commonly known as fatigue.[45] There are two main pathways, phosphagen and glycolysis (which includes the oxidative system as long as the oxygen supply is adequate). Even at rest, all the pathways are being used to a degree, and the percentage contribution of energy replenishment of each pathway depends on the rate, length of work time and required force development of the working muscles. It is only exercise that overloads the integrated cardiorespiratory system (pulmonary, cardiovascular

TRAINING THE DIFFERENT ATHLETIC COMPONENTS

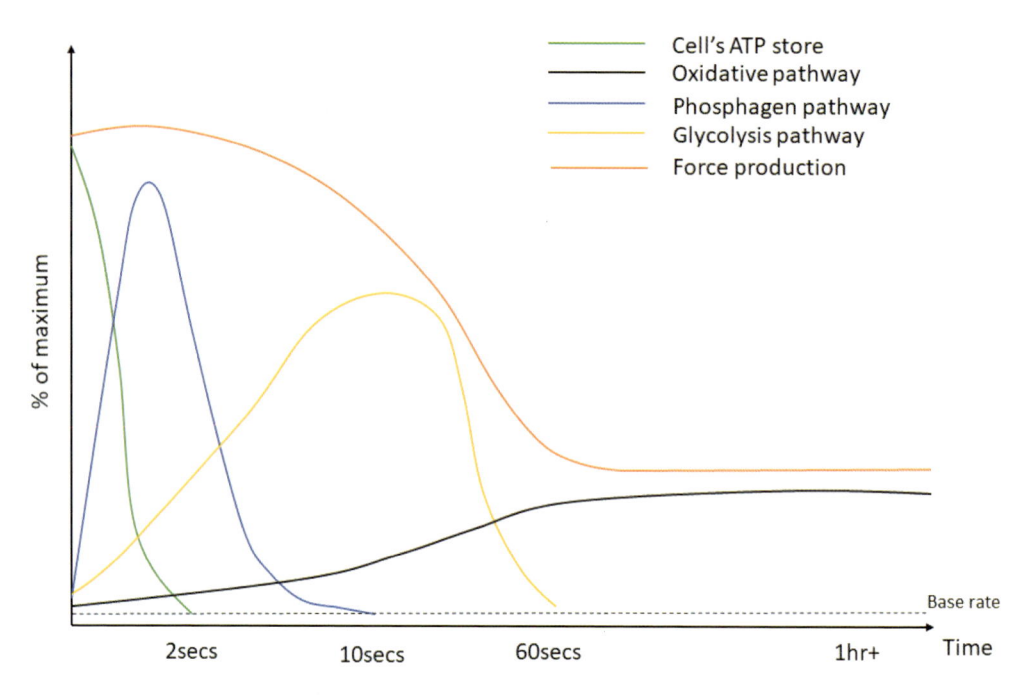

Fig. 8 Energy pathway contribution against force production over time for continuous exercise.

and neuromuscular) that will have a beneficial effect. This is why your current dance training is not having a positive effect on your cardiorespiratory fitness, as although you are dancing long hours the intensity is not enough to cause adaptations.[1,7]

Few forms of dance are continuous exercise and therefore dance generally falls under the umbrella of intermittent exercise. The ability of the energy production pathways to replenish the muscles' ATP stores between exercise/dance bouts depends on the length of the recovery period and the intensity of the dance bouts. The higher the intensity of dance bout, the longer the recovery period needed before you are able to replicate the same bout. Therefore, the work:rest ratio of interval training will not only challenge the ability of the energy pathways to produce energy for the exercise bout but also to improve recovery between bouts.

The oxidative system is vital to the recovery between the interval bouts and needs to be developed initially so that the subsequent interval training sessions can be beneficial. Steady-state training develops this foundation; the intensity should be moderate to high but not so high that you can't complete 20–30 minutes. There are several methods of determining intensity and these depend on the equipment available to you. The RPE scales, Fig. 4 in Chapter 2, provide a simple method of determining intensity, or heart rate zones if you have a heart rate monitor (Table 4). You don't need to do more than 30 minutes, as you are not trying to become an endurance athlete.

Once a good aerobic foundation has been developed, interval sessions can be incorporated. These have specific work:rest ratios according to the energy pathway you want to stress. Shorter recovery periods mean that the ATP stores are not fully recovered and therefore the intensity of the following bouts needs to be at a lower intensity to be able to complete them. A one-to-one ratio trains the oxidative pathway; a one-to-three ratio the glycolytic pathway, and

TRAINING THE DIFFERENT ATHLETIC COMPONENTS

$220 - age = HR_{max} \pm 12 b.min^{-1}$

$Oxidative\ Lower\ Training\ Heart\ Rate = HR_{max} \times 0.7$

$Oxidative\ Upper\ Training\ Heart\ Rate = HR_{max} \times 0.9$

For example

$220 - 22 = 198 b.min^{-1} (range: 188 - 210 b.min^{-1})$

$Oxidative\ Lower\ Training\ Heart\ Rate = 198 \times 0.7 = 139 b.min^{-1}\ (range: 132 - 146 b.min^{-1})$

$Oxidative\ Upper\ Training\ Heart\ Rate = 198 \times 0.9 = 178 b.min^{-1}\ (range: 169 - 187 b.min^{-1})$

Fig. 9 Calculating heart rate training zones.

Energy pathway	Training type	Overall duration	Training intensity	Recovery intensity	Interval duration
Oxidative	Continuous	20–30 minutes	70–90% HRmax 13–17 Borg Scale 5–8 Modified Borg		
Oxidative	Interval 1:1	20–30 minutes	85–90% HRmax 16–17 Borg Scale 7–8 Modified Borg	120 b.min^{-1} 11 Borg Scale 2 Modified Borg	2–3 min exercise 2–3 min recovery
Glycolytic (anaerobic)	Interval 1:3	20–30 minutes	90–100% HRmax 18–19 Borg Scale 9–10 Modified Borg	120 b.min^{-1} 11 Borg Scale 2 Modified Borg	30–100 sec exercise 90–300 sec recovery
Phosphagen (anaerobic)	Interval 1:5	15–20 minutes	100% HRmax 10 Borg Scale 10 Modified Borg	120 b.min^{-1} 11 Borg Scale 2 Modified Borg	10–15 sec exercise 50–75 sec recovery

Table 4 Training the cardiorespiratory pathways: intensity, duration and repetitions.

a one-to-five ratio the phosphagen pathway. As the recovery ratio periods get longer the actual exercise bouts gets shorter. Fig. 6 shows the length of time each pathway can maximally replenish energy; therefore, phosphagen training has bouts of 10–15 seconds, glycolytic training 30–100 seconds and aerobic training 2–3 minutes (Table 4).

What mode of activity?

As mentioned in Chapter 1, cardiorespiratory training has both central and peripheral (muscular) adaptations, therefore you need to be careful regarding the type of activity you choose to do. Ideally similar muscles that are engaged during dancing are preferable; therefore, running or the cross-trainer is better than rowing, which is better than cycling. Swimming has little transference at all, though it can be used as a recovery activity. Running often has a bad press, but it is a good form of activity as long as you start gradually and wear appropriate shoes. As running is in parallel (feet pointing forwards) there is increased engagement of the internal hip rotators which helps reduce the muscular imbalance around the hips caused from dancing in turnout. Also, because running emphasizes the stretch-shortening cycle there is a positive carryover to improving jump height. Initially there will be an increase in DOMS, particularly in the lower leg, if you are not used to running, but stretching and warm-down will reduce its effect.

If you are already doing a lot of jumping during dancing, a non-impact activity, such as the cross-trainer/stepper, or stationary bike, would be more appropriate to reduce the stress going through your body.

Frequency

The literature varies widely regarding the training frequencies required to cause adaptation. Depending on levels of initial fitness, 2–3 sessions a week are enough to have beneficial effects, though the American College of Sports Medicine recommends 5 sessions a week for the general population. For dancers we have found 2–3 sessions to be enough to cause a training effect, as you are already doing a lot of exercise,[10,11] but the intensity needs to be sufficient (*see* Table 4).

Progression

As you become fitter your heart rate or RPE will decrease if the training intensity stays the same. Thereby to maintain or improve your cardiorespiratory fitness you need to increase the training stress. This can be achieved by either increasing the intensity, duration or frequency of the training sessions. We recommend an increase in training intensity (speed or resistance), so it remains within the prescribed intensities rather than changing the frequency or duration of these sessions.

Target capacities

The most accurate method to calculate aerobic capacity is to have a maximal aerobic or VO_2max test, though we recognize few have access to such a test. Current research suggests a basic level of 50 $ml.kg^{-1}.min^{-1}$ for females and 60 $ml.kg^{-1}.min^{-1}$ for males (this is the amount of oxygen used per kilogram body weight per minute). Other tests include the dance aerobic fitness test for contemporary dance[46] and ballet;[47] for both of these tests heart rate is recorded at the end of each stage and the aim is to finish stage 5 with a heart rate 80 per cent of your maximum (*see* page 51).

Muscle Function

The overarching term 'muscle function' covers a wide range of muscle strength abilities. At its most basic, it refers to the number of contractions and the weight moved; how these two variables are manipulated will have widely differing effects. Some definitions that should be considered when planning interventions are the following:

- **Maximum strength** is the greatest force a muscle or group of muscles can generate during one movement, 1 repetition maximum or 1-RM. This is often used as the universal currency during training with different repetition maximum depending on the goal of the training: 10-RM for hypertrophy training or 15-RM for muscle endurance training.
- **Relative strength** is the relationship between a person's maximum strength and their body weight. It is often used as a goal-achievement target; for example, being able to squat 1.5BW (105kg for a dancer weighing 70kg).
- **General strength** is the strength of the whole body and is fundamental to furthering more specific strength training interventions. Depending on your training age, general strength can be the focus either as part of the preparatory phase's foundation training or it can be the sole focus for the first few years of supplemental training.

- **Specific strength** pertains to exercises that use the same motor patterns of muscle groups that are essential, in this instance, to dance. This type of training occurs after the foundation training.
- **Power** is the ability to generate force quickly and at high speeds and is essential to most dance genres. Ideally this needs to be developed after specific strength training.
- **Muscle endurance** is the ability to produce force through repetitive contraction over an extended period of time. This again preferably needs to be developed after specific strength training and is crucial to dance, particularly for the lower limbs.

What mode of resistance?

There is a wide range of ways of applying resistance to movements ranging from body weight to expensive machines. Each has its pros and cons which we will review, but we recognize that the decision of what modality to use is often dependent on access and availability.

Body weight

This is available for everyone and encompasses a wide variety of exercises. The exercises work by moving the body against gravity; changing the angle of the body, and therefore the body's centre of mass, can increase and decrease the resistance. Weighted vests can also be added to increase the resistance if need be. The use of ankle and wrist weights must be used with caution particularly with fast dynamic movements as they provide increased momentum and can cause muscle damage/tears in the opposing muscle (the one being stretched).

Weighted objects

As well as the weighted vests mentioned above, other objects include medicine balls, kettle bells, heavy ropes, sand-/water-filled balls, truck tyres. In all instances, resistance is achieved by moving the objects against gravity or the friction between object and floor.

Resistance bands

These are widely used but need to be incorporated with caution. When using them during a movement the speed of movement progressively decreases and resistance increases as the band is stretched. This means that often the muscle isn't challenged throughout its range of motion and is contrary to the muscle's force–length relationship. They are useful during rehabilitation exercises or to stimulate stabilizer muscle engagement during multi-joint movement (a band just above the knees during a squat action makes sure the hip stabilizers are engaged).

Weights machines

The gym is the bastion of weights machines, though there are home versions available. Resistance can be altered by repositioning a pin in the stack. Through the use of pulleys, cams and cables, pull-push/concentric/eccentric muscle actions are possible. There is a suggestion that these machines don't match a muscle's force–length relationship but recent developments in cam shape (this is an oddly shaped structure over which a cable runs around its perimeter and attaches to the machine arm) have improved this relationship.

Free weights

These – dumbbells and barbells – are considered the gold standard for strength training as they closely match the force–length relationship and mimic athletic movement patterns. The downside is that they require more skill to perform the exercises safely, but this also means that more muscles are engaged during the movement (stabilizers, synergists, co-agonists, etc.).

Isometric

This method of resistance applies to when the muscle force equals the resistance force, so that the limb and muscle don't change position. Isometric exercises are particularly useful when injured and a joint can't be taken through a full range of movement. The strength improvements usually have a beneficial effect 5–10-degrees each side of the isometric angle trained.

Training intensity

This refers to the resistance, load, or weight that you are using. Depending on the mode of resistance you are using (*see* above), how this is calculated will vary. Most S&C textbooks refer to this load as a percentage of the maximum amount you can lift (1 repetition max – 1-RM), but unless you have been training for quite a while, few people have the technical ability or experience to find their true 1-RM. In addition, your 1-RM will fluctuate depending on multiple factors such as nutritional status, recovery methods, sleep and so on. Another option is to experiment with the resistance until the last two repetitions of each exercise are a struggle. You will notice that a lot of 'serious' weight trainers carry a notebook around with them; this is just a record of what they did last time, so they don't have to try to remember not only the resistance but also the exercise. Different percentages of your maximal load help structure the training session according to its goals for example, muscular endurance, power or maximum strength (Fig. 10). Using body weight, resistance bands, or weighted objects will probably be limited to low- to medium-resistance intensities, whilst free weights and weight machines will be able to provide higher resistance intensities.

Repetitions and sets

The number of repetitions (reps) you can do is linked to the resistance load selected. Although Fig. 10 provides a rough idea of the number of repetitions that can be carried out there can be quite a range depending on your training status, sex, muscle mass engaged, and actual exercise being undertaken. The number of sets will also depend on the above variables. You should incorporate 1–2 warm-up sets at a lower resistance intensity before starting the training sets; these will prepare the movement patterns (neuromuscular pathways) before the increased load is applied. The number of training sets generally varies between 2 and 4; doing more isn't necessary as long as the resistance load is correct. The important aspect is quality, not quantity!

As indicated in Fig. 10 the number of repetitions chosen has a direct effect on specific physiological adaptations. Higher number of repetitions, with the corresponding low-intensity load, promotes muscular endurance as it engages the slow twitch fibres and promotes fatigue resistance through similar peripheral adaptations as aerobic fitness training. As one of the goals is fatigue resistance, the rest between sets should be minimal (1–2 minutes) but not too little so that the training reps are compromised. Power training is best

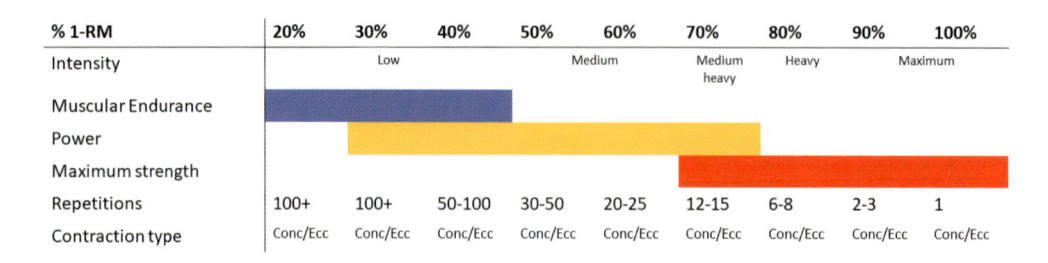

% 1-RM	20%	30%	40%	50%	60%	70%	80%	90%	100%
Intensity		Low			Medium	Medium heavy	Heavy		Maximum
Muscular Endurance									
Power									
Maximum strength									
Repetitions	100+	100+	50-100	30-50	20-25	12-15	6-8	2-3	1
Contraction type	Conc/Ecc	Conc/Ecc	Conc/Ecc	Conc/Ecc	Conc/Ecc	Conc/Ecc	Conc/Ecc	Conc/Ecc	Conc/Ecc

Fig. 10 Training intensity in relationship to training goals.

developed through low repetition regimens and longer recovery periods, as the focus is on neuromuscular development and increasing the rate of force development. The resistance load needs to be low to medium, so the speed of movement isn't compromised. The rest:work ratio is very important in strength training; if the rest period is short (around 1 minute) depending on the training adaptation wanted there may be hypertrophic adaptations (get bigger in size), while longer rest periods (2 minutes +) may promote neuromuscular changes. It is often the training load that dictates the time under tension and rest intervals and therefore this needs to be selected carefully to make sure you achieve your desired goals.

Training volume and progression

This is quantified by the amount lifted; for each exercise calculate the resistance load (kg, body weight, etc.), multiply with the number of reps and multiply with the number of sets and then sum up the subtotals from each exercise for the grand total. The use of the grand total will allow progression loads to be calculated and planned. The volume should be increased 5–10 per cent per week during a training phase with an emphasis on increasing the resistance load rather than increasing the number of repetitions.

FLEXIBILITY

Not all stretching is the same
Dancers are renowned for their flexibility, but there is quite a difference between genres regarding the range of movement (ROM) required at different joints. It is not just about having a large ROM but also being able to use the available range safely and in a controlled manner; strength is therefore an integral part of flexibility training. Being hyperflexible is just as much an injury risk as being inflexible, so you often don't need to be really flexible in every joint, in every direction, just those relevant to your genre.

Stretching is obviously the main way that these ROMs are achieved, but not all methods of stretching are equal and different techniques should be used at different times. Each muscle has two main feedback mechanisms that provide feedback regarding their length and the amount of strain they are under. A muscle's length is monitored by the muscle spindle, a stretchable intrafusal fibre that runs the length of each muscle. At a muscle's resting length a slow steady feedback signal is sent back to the brain; when a muscle is stretched, the feedback signals increase according to how far the muscle is being stretched (the greater the stretch the more signals). When a muscle is being contracted the signals get less or stop. It is through this feedback mechanism that we know where each limb is without having to look at it for confirmation. The other important feedback we receive is from the Golgi Tendon Organ (GTO), this measures the amount of strain or force that is going through the tendon; generally the feedback signals increase as the muscle is contracting under load.

The stretch reflex
This has a dynamic and a static component. The GTO is responsible for the dynamic component: it sends rapid signals in response to the sudden increase in muscle length and only lasts a short period of time. The muscle spindle provides the static component, with signals increasing in frequency as the muscle increases in length. During a rapid stretch, like a fast, uncontrolled grande battement, both the GTO and the muscle spindle fire rapidly and the stretch reflex can cause the muscle to contract to protect it.

The lengthening reaction
This is also known as autogenic inhibition; the GTO measures change in tension in the tendon, and when this exceeds a certain threshold, the lengthening reaction is triggered, causing the

muscle to relax by inhibiting contraction. The lengthening reaction is possible because the GTO signal overrides muscle spindle signals trying to cause muscle contraction. Holding a stretch for a prolonged period of time, over 30 seconds, engages the lengthening reaction, thus helping the stretched muscles to relax. It is easier to lengthen a muscle when it is not trying to contract.

What happens when you stretch?

The first increase in muscle length when stretching is the decrease in overlap between the actin and myosin filaments in the muscle fibrils (Chapter 1). When the sarcomeres are fully lengthened, further elongation is achieved by stretching the connective tissue. As the stretch tension increases, the collagen fibres realign themselves along the line of tension. This helps regain muscle range of movement post injury, as the collagen in scar tissue is disorganized. But when we start to stretch, only some fibres lengthen and others remain at their resting length; therefore, the length a muscle can be elongated depends on the number of muscle fibres actually being stretched. Part of flexibility training is 'learning' to allow more fibres to be stretched.

How is increased range of movement achieved?

This is still under debate, though there are two main schools of thought. The first is muscle fibres increase in length by increasing the number of sarcomeres. There is evidence that this might occur from animal studies, though whether something similar occurs in human muscles isn't known. The other is called stretch tolerance; this refers to how we get used to the feeling of a stretch. Initially the stretch may have an 8/10 pain rating, but over time this sensation decreases to 4/10 as you get used to it.

Stretching position

To stretch a muscle, it needs to be totally relaxed and therefore the position we use is very important. Standing hamstring stretches, with the leg being stretched on the barre for instance, actually means the hamstring is under tension as it is also providing support and therefore can't fully relax. Therefore, if instead you lie on your back and then flex the leg towards you, the amount of tension in the hamstrings is reduced. The tension is further reduced if you support your leg with your arms. Taking time to make sure the muscle being stretched is under as little tension as possible is important to optimize the stretch.

Duration

Depending on the type of stretch being employed (*see* next section), generally a stretch should be held for between 1 and 2 minutes, as this will engage the lengthening reaction. Some research has shown equal increases in range of movement for stretches held for 30–60 seconds; therefore, there is little benefit in holding a stretch for long periods of time.

Intensity

There is a growing body of evidence that moderate-intensity stretching (5–6/10) is more beneficial for recovery post-exercise than high-intensity stretching.[37,48] Remember this isn't the range of movement but the feeling of intensity in the muscle being stretched. One of the problems of moderate-intensity stretching is that it doesn't feel it is doing anything and there is a tendency to want to push harder, but high-intensity stretching can cause muscle damage.[49] High-intensity stretching (above 8/10) should only be employed as part of a warm-up protocol when the muscle has been warmed up.

Order

We all like to stretch what we are good at, but this often means the muscles that are the most flexible just increase their range of movement to the detriment of tighter muscles. Therefore, it is good to work on areas of tightness first but also to think of muscle's kinetic chains – for instance, the calves and glutes should be stretched before the hamstrings.

Types of stretch

There are a number of different stretching methods that can be applied to any muscle. The important thing is to select the correct method for the situation you are in or the goal you are working towards. The stretches utilized during a warm-up are different from those used during a warm-down or to increase range of movement. There has been some research suggesting that passive stretching can affect muscle power, and this is the case if a jump is carried out immediately after a passive stretch; but this is rarely the case in real life. It is proposed that holding a passive stretch for a long period of time, more than 1 minute, either affects the blood flow to the muscle or impinges its motor neurons, thereby reducing the muscle's ability to generate force. During a warm-up, whether for dance or supplemental fitness training, passive stretching can be implemented but subsequent movements need to be dynamic to negate any possible negative effects. There are two types of warm-down: a short one between classes/rehearsals during the training day or a longer one at the end of the training day. The short warm-down is about recovery between training sessions. The stretches employed during this warm-down are about reminding a muscle of its full range of movement; they need to take the muscle through its full range of movement but held for just 6–10 seconds. This type of stretch resets the muscle ready for the next session. The focus of the long warm-down, at the end of the day, is on preventing or reducing the effect of the day's exercise. One of the negative effects of exercise, especially impact movements such as jumping, is the formation of micro-scarring on the muscle's epimysium. The collagen tissue in scar tissue is random in direction and therefore contrary to the muscle's direction of elongation; stretching helps align these fibres, thereby reducing the effect of exercise. These stretches need to be held for a longer period of time, around 1 minute, which engages the lengthening reaction.

Passive stretching

This involves stretching a muscle by using an external force to lengthen it. For instance, to stretch the hamstrings someone else moves the leg into flexion and supports the leg during the stretch. This could also be yourself, if you use a strap or band to move the leg, and do not engage your hip flexors. This can be integrated into a warm-up as long as other mobilization activities and dynamic movements occur subsequently; within this scenario stretches should be held for just 30 seconds. Passive stretching can be used as part of a warm-down and to increase range of movement; in both these situations, the stretch needs to be held for longer, around 1 minute.

Active stretching

This involves using an agonist muscle to move a limb, so the antagonist muscle is stretched. This type of stretch utilizes reciprocal inhibition, a neuromuscular phenomenon, that causes the opposite muscle in a pairing to relax when the other is contracting. Using the hamstring as an example, by engaging the hip flexors and quadricep muscles to cause straight leg hip flexion, the hamstrings are inhibited and therefore can be stretched. This method of stretching is ideal for a warm-up as it engages the agonist muscle and starts to prepare the body for functional movement.

Dynamic stretching

Unlike passive and active stretching, where the muscle is held in a static position for a period of time, dynamic stretching involves taking a muscle through its range of movement at a moderate speed in a controlled manner.

A grande battement is a prime example of dynamic stretching. This obviously requires the muscle to be warm beforehand and therefore should occur towards the end of a warm-up. It has a neuromuscular component in that it prepares the muscle to work eccentrically; the use of moderate speed also starts to prepare the muscle for the faster movements experienced during dance or supplemental training.

Ballistic stretching

This is a faster version of dynamic stretching and resembles the fast limb speeds during jumping. It can be incorporated into a warm-up if the subsequent movements are going to be fast. Because there is a big eccentric component to the stretch (the muscle acting as a brake towards its full range of movement) it can cause DOMS and possible injury. Even though this type of stretching has an increased risk, when incorporated correctly it leads to improved physical performance.

Proprioceptive neuromuscular facilitation (PNF)

This is an advanced method of stretching initially developed for rehabilitation; ideally it requires a partner. PNF can put increased stress on the muscles as it overrides some of its protective mechanisms, possibly increasing the risk of injury. It involves both stretching and contracting a muscle to increase its range of movement. It isn't necessary to apply maximum force during the contraction or stretch phase to achieve results and intensities around 6/10 have been shown to be beneficial. One of the main PNF techniques is stretch–contract–stretch; this is when a muscle is initially stretched to the end point of range of movement, the stretched muscle is then isometrically contracted for 5–6 seconds against an immovable object or partner at this end range before the contracted muscle is then relaxed and a controlled stretch is applied for a further 20–30 seconds. The stretch can be repeated two to four times with a 30-second rest in between.

Aggressive stretching

This type of stretching is ideal between training sessions or dance classes/rehearsals. Often, immediately after a hard session, a muscle becomes stiff with a reduced range of movement. An aggressive stretch aims to take the muscle to its full range of movement and hold it there in a static stretch for 5–6 seconds to 'reset' it.

PLYOMETRIC AND AGILITY TRAINING

Plyometrics consists of exercises such as hopping, skipping and jumping that are focused on helping you jump higher and move more quickly; agility on the other hand is the ability to change direction quickly. Both of these are fundamental skills for dancers but are rarely trained specifically. Dance class has a lot of jumps, but the emphasis is on the aesthetic and not how to jump. A study recorded the jump height of male and female ballet dancers from eleven years old to professional; male dancers increased their jump height by 33 per cent between the ages of eleven to eighteen, whilst female dancers reported just a 6 per cent increase. In comparison athletes were reported to increase vertical jump height by 41 per cent and 24 per cent respectively over the same age range. Professional male ballet dancers recorded a mean jump height of 52cm and females 37cm; 62 per cent and 67 per cent increase compared to the heights achieved during pre-professional training. This difference between pre-professional and professional dancers, particularly in female dancers, could be due to a lack of emphasis on jumping big in their training whilst at school, coupled with a lack of specific physical fitness training.

Prior to plyometric training, you should undergo a period of strength training to prepare the body for the high-intensity exercise; strength training will increase the strength of the tendons, muscles and joints.

TRAINING THE DIFFERENT ATHLETIC COMPONENTS

Fundamental to plyometric training is moving at maximum speed; training at submaximal speeds and intensities will produce submaximal results. This again highlights the importance of specificity in training. The use of ankle weights and sand training might increase the intensity of the exercise, but they slow down movement and therefore the benefits are lost. Jumping on a foam pad is good for training ankle stability and control but not for increasing jump height.

Plyometric training is focused on causing adaptation to two specific and linked systems. Firstly, mechanical or kinetic energy: this is produced when a muscle, or more importantly its tendon, is rapidly stretched. The energy is generated by the stretching of the series elastic component (SEC) of the muscle and tendon (Chapter 1) during an eccentric muscle action; if a muscle begins a concentric action immediately after the eccentric action the stored energy is released, allowing the SEC to contribute to the total force production. If the muscle doesn't contract immediately or the eccentric phase is too long (for example, a deep plié) then the stored energy is lost as heat. The neurophysiological system is the second system and involves training the muscle's potentiation. When a muscle is rapidly stretched (as monitored by the muscle spindles – Chapter 1), the stretch reflex is stimulated causing a reflexive muscle contraction. This is the basis of plyometric training: muscle spindles are stimulated by the rapid muscle stretch and this response potentiates, increases, the activity on the muscle thereby increasing the contractile force of the muscle.

The stretch-shortening cycle is fundamental to our locomotion and comprises three phases: the eccentric phase, the amortization phase and the concentric phase – or, in other words, landing, stance and take-off. The eccentric phase is the pre-loading phase with the storage of kinetic energy and the stimulation of the stretch reflex. The amortization phase is the time between the end of the eccentric phase to the initiation of the concentric muscle contraction. The longer this phase the more kinetic energy is lost, so the aim of plyometric training is to minimize the amortization time. The rate of the stretch is very important: the faster the stretch the greater the muscle recruitment and activity during the concentric phase. This is obviously a difficulty within dance, when the speed of jumps is determined by the music and the technique of 'going through your foot' on landing increases the amortization period.

Jumping is a multi-joint movement with the main joints being the ankle, knee and hip. These don't all contribute equally to the power production during a jump and recent research suggests most of the power is generated around the ankle joint in dance jumps. This is in contrast to the majority of sportspeople who utilize the knee and hip as the main power generators; this is potentially due to the different body position that dancers and athletes use when jumping. The upright torso position that dancers assume possibly reduces the contribution of the hip and to a lesser extent the knee. Rarely are all the joints/muscles used optimally and the use of different plyometric exercises can be used to engage underused muscles within jump sequence. Although the ankle joint is possibly the main contributor of power, the hip complex should also be focused on, especially movements that engage the posterior chain (glutes and hamstrings).

Recovery is a vital component of plyometric training; because of the emphasis on rapid eccentric loading, DOMS (Chapter 2) is a regular outcome and therefore there should be 48–72 hours' recovery between sessions. It also needs to be incorporated carefully into your wider dance schedule so that it doesn't compromise rehearsals or performances.

Adolescents can benefit from plyometric training though the training plans need to be adapted. In pre-pubescent children the growth plates are still open and high-intensity loading can cause premature closing of these plates. Low-intensity exercises though will have beneficial neuromuscular, physiological and anatomical adaptations; therefore, the focus should be on the quality and control of the movements to develop the techniques they will use when they are older.

Dance covers a multitude of genres and movement patterns and current choreography often blends across these. Therefore, being agile – the ability to change direction whilst maintaining good body control – is essential for a dancer. Agility is often referred to as a person's coordinative abilities; these abilities are considered to be most trainable during late childhood to early adolescence, which coincides with the time when young dancers start to do more classes. This might seem a good thing but often the early specialization promoted within the dance world actually limits a dancer's development. Their movement patterns are limited to patterns determined by a few dance genres and the transferability is diminished with the limitation of movement experiences often allowed during pre-professional dance training. Professional dancers are now required to carry out movement patterns (choreography) outside of their main skills set (genre) and an underlying agility, developed throughout their late childhood to late adolescence, to be able to move in a fast, controlled manner helps with this transition.

Fundamental to agility is the ability to control your centre of gravity whilst changing direction, usually in several planes of movement simultaneously. Dance consists of multi-dimensional movement and agility training is essential for a dancer. The key to agility training is the maintenance of speed when shifting the body's centre of gravity and exercises should focus on rapid changes in direction. One of the main effects of agility training is an increase in body control and how to make minimal postural adjustments to maintain balance during extreme movements.

It might seem that plyometric and agility training is superfluous for dancers as they train skills integral to dance. By developing these attributes beyond the demands required by dance, it means that when dancing you will be working at a lower percentage of your maximum capabilities and will therefore be less likely to become fatigued. Plyometric and agility prescription is similar to other interventions with reps, sets, rest and progression. Because of the high intensity and loading during these training sessions, this type of training should be undertaken when fresh (not fatigued) and after a good warm-up.

Plyometric Training

Intensity

Factors that determine intensity include points of contact (single-leg exercises place more stress on the muscles, tendons and joints than double-leg exercises); speed (the greater the speed the greater the intensity); body weight (the heavier the person the greater the stress on the person's tendons, joints and muscles – weighted vests can be used to increase an exercise's intensity); centre of gravity (the use of boxes to jump/drop off). The maximal height of the box used for depth jumps will vary according to the experience and strength of the person, but generally it ranges from 41cm (beginners) to 110cm (highly trained). If the height you choose is too high the load experienced may be too great to control effectively; this increases the likelihood of injury but also means the amortization period becomes too long and therefore the purpose of the exercise is defeated.

Reps and sets

Even though you have been jumping as part of your dance, you should initially consider yourself a beginner when you start to do plyometric training as the actions and forces are different to what you are used to. Fundamental to plyometric training is the quality of the training rather than the quantity, so it is better to

TRAINING THE DIFFERENT ATHLETIC COMPONENTS

maximize every repetition than do more poor-quality repetitions. The volume of exercise is usually expressed as the total number of repetitions, or contacts, performed during the training session; beginners would start with 80–100 contacts, those moderately trained 100–120 and highly trained 120–140. Most exercises should be limited to 8–10 repetitions and 2–3 sets; the rest between sets will vary according to the exercises selected. Low- to moderate-intensity exercises can use a 1:5 work:rest ratio but for high-intensity exercises a longer rest period can be incorporated to maximize repetition performance.

Progression

Progress should start with low to moderate volumes of low-intensity plyometrics, followed by low to moderate volumes of moderate intensity and finally low to moderate volumes of high-intensity exercises. A session for a moderate to highly trained person can include a variety of exercises that range between low and high-intensity loading depending on their requirements. When moving from low to moderate or moderate to high-intensity exercises you should decrease the volume of your contacts to allow your body to adapt to the increased load. As mentioned previously, the body can cope with approximately 10 per cent increase in load a week, in this instance other jumping activities need to be taken into account. If you are doing a lot of jumping during class, rehearsals and performances, the number of contacts during plyometric training should be decreased but not ceased. The important aspect is quality not quantity!

AGILITY TRAINING

Intensity

Exercises should be started at a slow to moderate pace until adequate control is achieved. There are two reasons for this: firstly, to make sure the limb alignment and movement patterning is correct; and secondly, because the braking phase of the acceleration-braking-acceleration requires the muscles to work eccentrically, and an increase in movement speed increases the eccentric action and therefore muscle damage. Also, the greater the change in direction of your body's centre of mass the increased loading of the braking muscles. This is not necessarily just a linear change in direction but can also include moving down and up from the floor and interacting with other dancers. The main change in intensity is the change in speed of the activity and the magnitude of the change in direction.

Repetitions and sets

Similar to plyometric training, the focus for agility training is the quality of the practice, not the quantity. Exercise repetitions and sets should be kept to around 5–6 repetitions and 2–3 sets. As most of the exercises are timed, the rest periods are easy to calculate using a 1:5 work:rest ratio. There should be little fluctuation in the repetition times (around 10 per cent of the average time); if times do drop considerably, either increase the rest period or stop the training altogether.

Progression

As mentioned in the intensity section, progression can be an increase in speed or magnitude of direction change. Often the training session doesn't feel hard, as the effects aren't felt until the following day, so there is a tendency to want to do too much in a session. Plan your progressions, monitor how your body feels the next day, and keep to your schedule.

CORE TRAINING

This has been a major focus in everybody's training programme for a long time, as this area, the lumbo-pelvic-hip complex, links the upper and lower body and provides stabilization to the spine. The muscles include the hip adductors, gluteus medius, gluteus minimus, gluteus maximus, erector spinae, rectus abdominis, hamstrings, piriformis, ilio-psoas, transverse abdominis, multifidus, quadratus lumborum, pelvic floor, diaphragm, and internal and external obliques. The muscles of the core act as a corset between the ribs and pelvis and need to be able to allow the body to carry out its functional movement patterns whilst providing power, strength and stabilization. The continuum ranges from core rigidity during lifts and jumps to fast, dynamic twisting actions seen in hip-hop and breakin'; but simply the core provides stability, lateral flexion, rotation, and flexion and extension. Any activity can cause an imbalance within the core musculature, particularly if there are repetitious movements on one side of the body – for example, the use of the right leg as the main gesture leg or always spiralling in one direction.

Supplemental core training should aim to maintain a balance between the muscular and also develop the core's ability to cope with foreseen and unforeseen demands. Training is often at the end of a workout and consists of flexion-extension exercises such as crunches or 100s, which rarely mimic the movement patterns required for dance. These exercises don't address the requirements for developing a strong, powerful stable link between the upper and lower body. There are calls for core training to be moved to the start of training, rather than a last-minute add on, due to its importance.[50] Initial training should use isolation exercises to improve core muscle activation before more integrated functional exercises are used.[51] The latter are fundamental as they provide co-ordination of these muscles within whole body movements, for example the erector spinae need to be trained in conjunction with the glutes and hamstrings as part of the posterior kinetic chain. The chosen exercises shouldn't be limited to movements when lying on the ground but become more functional and use standing, bridging (feet and shoulders touching the floor) and quadruped (hands and knees/toes) positions, thereby mimicking the movements carried out during dance.

Engaging the right muscles is an essential aspect of core training and the hollowing or drawing-in of the core, fundamental to Pilates movements, means that the transverse abdominis is engaged rather than the external obliques. Research has shown that just prior to any limb movement the transverse abdominis contracts and, along with the internal obliques, are the only muscles attached to the thoracolumbar fascia thereby preventing spine flexion (they act as a weight belt). Engagement of the transverse abdominis does not prevent movement from occurring, therefore hollowing followed by rotational movements will help to make sure that the right muscles are engaged. If you are using your internal and/or external obliques to achieve the hollowing effect, any rotational or lateral flexion movement won't be possible or will be very limited. Bracing is slightly different and is when you want your core area to be rigid. This is needed during whole body strength movements such as deadlifts; you need to engage your transverse abdominis and internal and external obliques to make the whole area rigid.

The pelvic floor is another integral part of the core musculature and is often overlooked by men and young women, the latter only becoming truly aware of it postpartum. The pelvic floor muscles form a 'hammock' between the pubic bone and coccyx (front to back) and the two ischial tuberosities (left to right). Obviously through these muscles run the urethra and anus as well as the vagina for women. Contracting the pelvic floor lifts the internal organs of the pelvis and tightens the openings of the urethra, anus and vagina. These muscles can be trained like any other and initially may require focused training, before making sure they are engaged during more complex movements.

An aspect of core training that has been very well developed in sport is 'bracing'. This increases the internal pressure of the abdominal area by co-contracting the deep and superficial abdominals, pulling up the pelvic floor and pushing down the diaphragm. The result is that the area between the ribs and pelvis becomes rigid. This is useful when carrying out maximal exertions or lifting a weight, or dancer, above your head, but for maximal benefits the muscular needs to be developed initially.

Exercise selection

Core programmes focus too much on flexion-extension exercises and not enough on lateral flexion and stabilization movements; we also often get stuck doing the same exercises all the time, when variety is the spice of life, especially for your core. The stability/Swiss/Pilates ball has become a major component of programmes, but it is often introduced too quickly. Stability training should start on the floor and only progress to an unstable surface when you have developed the correct movement patterns and conditioning. Fast movements and standing exercises need to be incorporated, as well as the usual slow controlled actions, to prepare the body for dance. Medicine ball training (fast movements) allows actions to be more dance-specific by bridging the gap between conventional core exercise movements and dance. They incorporate power development and whole-body, functional movement as the exercises require the transfer of power from the floor, through the legs, the torso and eventually out through the arms whilst the muscles are contracting at speeds similar to that encountered during dance. One of the major limitations of medicine ball work is it requires space and often a solid surface to throw the ball against. You also don't feel the 'burn' (usually felt during core training) until the next day. Standing core exercises usually use a cable-column machine; these are expensive and the exercises, such as the chop and lift, are not easy to learn, but the movements are more functional, and they allow the progression from stabilization exercises to dynamic resisted exercises.

Intensity

After foundational development of the core muscular with traditional low-intensity core exercises, intensity and complexity can be developed using stability balls, medicine balls and cable-column machines. The latter two modes of training can increase intensity easily by either using a heavier medicine ball or more weight on the cables. Remember the core is also being trained when you do other training, especially weight training; exercises such as the deadlift and squat put a lot of force through the core.

Repetitions and sets

As with all movement patterns, as soon as form or technique is lost, have a rest. Generally, for low-intensity core exercises sets of 20–25 repetitions are fine; instead of maybe doing 3 sets of 25 crunches with a short rest in between each set, you can change the type of exercise each set, which will delay localized fatigue. For the high-intensity exercises, a lower number of repetitions (10–12) and a longer rest between sets is required to make sure form is maintained.

Progression

Progression is often perceived as just doing more repetitions until the 'burn' is felt. This method just improves core endurance and unless correct technique and muscle engagement is maintained throughout the repetitions, muscle imbalances will start to develop. It is a good idea to mix the movement patterns up as much as possible, as this will also cause an overload to be developed. Remember a

TRAINING THE DIFFERENT ATHLETIC COMPONENTS

six-pack is not a sign of a well-developed core, just low body fat!

Balance and Stability

We use feedback from our internal and external sensory systems to maintain our centre of gravity (usually around our belly button) over our base of support (the body part(s) in contact with the floor) by minute, rapid muscle contractions. These mechanisms are utilized during both movement and standing in place. Just lifting an arm or leg requires you to make adjustments so you don't fall over, and all movement requires becoming unstable, moving your centre of gravity beyond your base of support, before recovering, usually by moving a leg, to regain stability. Postural stability refers to the amount you can move your centre of gravity away from your base of support before you fall over or have to change your base of support. Postural control is your ability to maintain control during movement and allows you to utilize momentum and limb movement to prevent falling over, unless that is the point of the movement. The travel observed during multiple pirouettes or fouetté turns relates to postural control – the greater the travel the less control. We all have different abilities based on numerous factors such as body shape, foot size, type of shoes worn and experience, and we can train these skills to improve our abilities.

Some aspects of stability training are covered in the core training section and along the same vein, every activity can be adapted to increase the stability component of the exercise by gradually increasing the instability of the surface; this is sometimes referred to as functional training. Practising landing techniques or 'sticking' a landing is ideal preparation prior to jump or plyometric training but can be taken further by gradually increasing the softness of the surface you are landing on, e.g. landing on a foam mat rather than the floor, and then landing on one leg instead of two. This then can be progressed to faster dynamic movements such as multiple linear hops developing into multidirectional hops. Chest training might start with a fixed weights machine before progressing to a free-weights bar to dumbbells to press-ups using a Bosu ball or stability ball. An obvious important factor is to train your non-dominant side as well, as this side often gets overlooked. The focus of the training is on challenging your movement control, so it is less about increasing the resistance/force being exerted but possibly either increasing the instability of the surface or the speed of the movement – but not both at the same time.

Rest, Hydration and Nutrition

These factors are as essential to training as the training sessions themselves and should be planned into your schedules. The theory behind what happens during recovery is covered in Chapter 2 but the body, and in particular the muscles, need a period of rest after training to allow for adaptation. Sleep is the most important aspect of recovery, and it is the quality of sleep that is important; it is during deep sleep that muscle repair is optimized. Evidence suggests that we need 8 hours' sleep a night; obviously each individual requires different amounts, but one thing is agreed upon: we need at least 1 hour of deep sleep. Monitoring how you feel when you wake up is a good method of determining if you need more: feeling fuzzy, fatigued, or not quite 'with it' is an easy indicator that more sleep is needed. Power naps during the day are wonderful but not always possible. Finding somewhere for a quiet 15-minute snooze can be revitalizing but also requires practice and access to a quiet place. Nutrition will be covered in more detail in Chapter 11, but in summary, food is our energy to fuel all your activities during the day. It is better to eat for what you are about to do, rather than for what you have done. It requires planning, both for what you are going to eat and also when you are going to have it.

4 SCREENING AND PROGRAMME DESIGN

Where do you start when deciding to include supplemental training in your schedule? What should you focus on? How do you decide what is more important than something else? How do you fit it in when you are already busy? We will attempt to answer these questions in this chapter and provide some guidance on how to keep it simple, straightforward, and time efficient.

NEEDS ANALYSIS

Butler[52] developed a process called Performance Profiling that makes a good construct to help you understand what are you requiring your body to do when you dance (Fig. 11). There are no right or wrong answers as it is based on your own perceptions, but it will allow you to think more deeply on what has often become automatic. Don't focus on skills but the underlying physical abilities. The first stage is to identify 10–20 characteristics/abilities you think the ultimate/ideal dancer should possess and then rate each one out of ten as to their importance. This doesn't mean that each characteristic/ability is 10/10 as not each will have the same importance. The second stage is to (honestly) rate yourself against these characteristics. The dif-

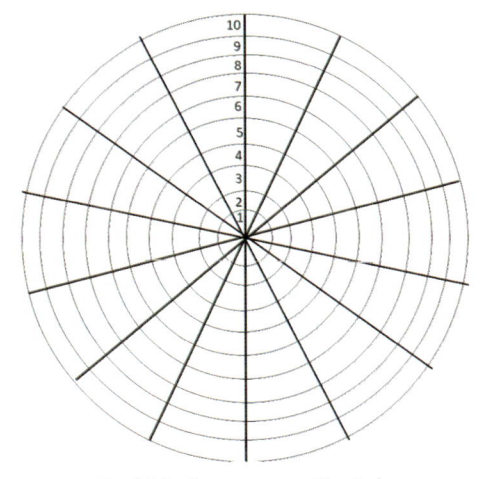

Fig. 11 Performance profile circle.

SCREENING AND PROGRAMME DESIGN

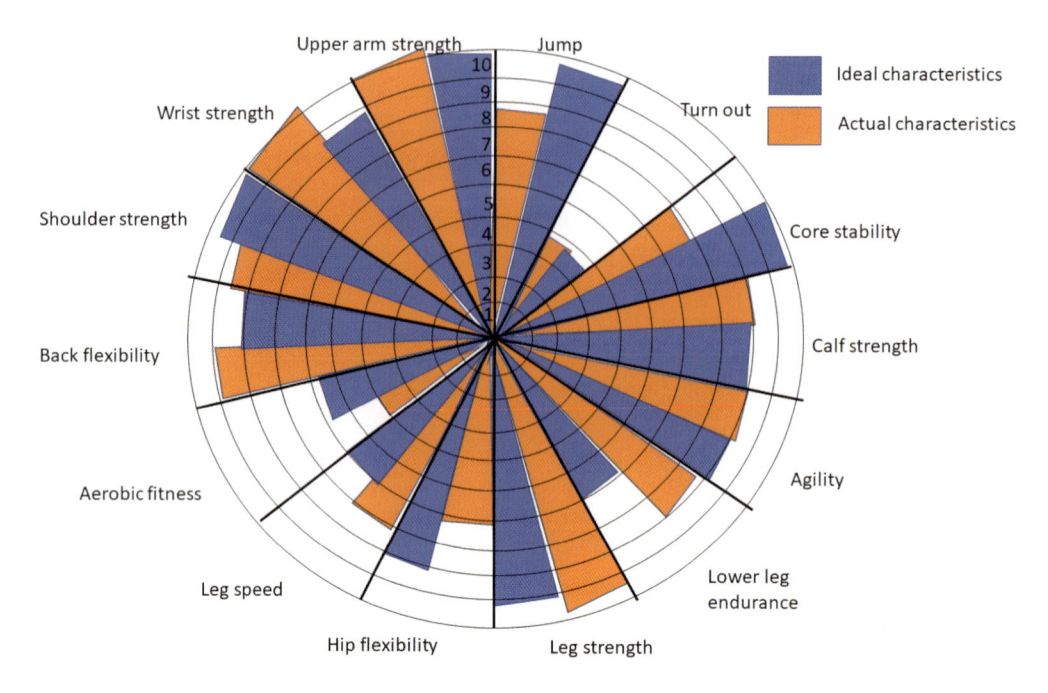

Fig. 12 An example of how the performance profile can be completed.

ference between the stage ratings provides an indication of characteristics/abilities that need developing; Fig. 12 is a hypothetical example.

The same process can be used to compare the foundation needs or general requirements of your dance genre to the performance demands (your next performance, show, competition or battle). Select 10–20 abilities required for performance and again rate each one out of 10; obviously there is going to be some overlap of characteristics/abilities with the first version. It is also important to remember that the characteristics/abilities could change with each performance as roles or choreography change. Next to these, rate how well these characteristics are developed during class or training. Again, the difference between these two ratings provides an idea of the supplemental training needed to bridge the gap between training and performance.

Some other things to think about when developing your dance needs analysis include (but are not limited to):

- Is it continuous movement or is it stop and start?
- Is the intensity pretty constant or is it forever changing with periods of really intense exercise followed by easier periods or periods off stage?
- How long do you have to dance for in one period, in a class or performance or in a day?
- How many jumps do you do in your training compared with a performance?
- Are you going to have to lift/support/catch someone?
- Does the movement/choreography emphasize one side of the body more than the other or a specific movement repetition?
- Is the movement fast or slow, controlled or dynamic?
- Are there a lot of de-accelerating actions (landing from jumps, rapid changes in direction)?

The above methods will provide you with an idea of where you are currently, the demands

SCREENING AND PROGRAMME DESIGN

of what you want to prepare for, and the areas that need developing to meet those demands. The limitation of this method is that it is subjective and based on your own perceptions, and it is also beneficial to supplement this with some objective data. It is the difference between 'I think I am jumping higher' to 'I'm jumping 5cm higher'; this can make a world of difference when it comes to goal-setting, as it will let you know when you have achieved it – this has an enormous motivating effect on future training sessions and goal achievements.

Do-It-Yourself Physical Fitness Screen

We have provided you with a range of different tests that we have organized into the different physical fitness categories. You don't need to do all of them but select the most appropriate ones for the areas of physical fitness you are trying to develop. That said, when you first start it is a good idea to do one or two tests in each category as this will give you a starting point and will also allow a comparison with your Needs Analysis results. This will see if your perceptions of your fitness levels are close to comparable data from other dancers. This can be a bit of a reality check but rather than de-motivating you, you should use the information to drive you forward. We have tried to provide as much comparable data as possible from other dancers, but where there isn't any information available, we have used our own clinical experience to provide analogous data.

Balance
These tests should be done on both legs to see if you have any bilateral differences. It is quite normal that one leg will be better than the other, particularly in theatrical dance genres where there is often an emphasis on the right leg as the main gesture leg, meaning the left leg is superior at balance.

Romberg test (stork balance test)
This is a very simple test based on how long (time) you can keep the position before losing balance or shifting your stance foot. Start standing upright with your arms folded against your chest, then close your eyes. As you lift one leg off the ground the time should start; the lifted leg should not be in contact with your stance leg but remain bent slightly. You should try to remain upright in this position as long as possible without moving the stance leg or wafting your arms around to maintain balance (Fig. 13). Repeat on the other leg. It might be a good idea to repeat 2 or 3 times on each leg.

Most reported criteria suggest a target time of 2 minutes; holding beyond this time provides no greater benefit, though I have had dancers last over 8 minutes. Also, you should

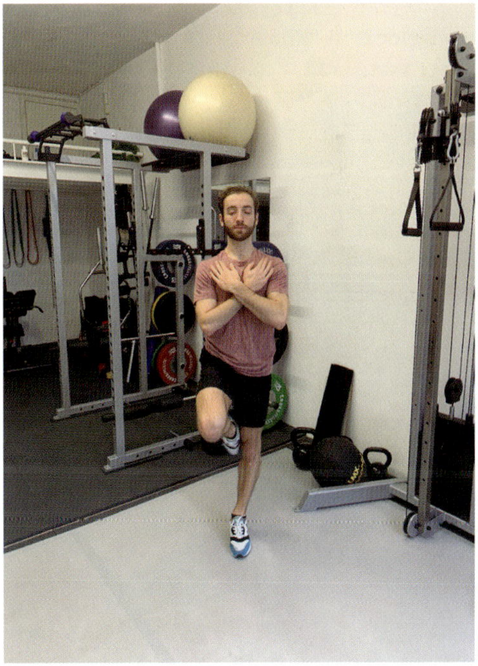

Fig. 13 Balance position for the Romberg Test.

SCREENING AND PROGRAMME DESIGN

look for similar abilities between the legs with no more than a 10 per cent difference in the time held.

Star excursion test

Initially you need to set up the test as indicated in Fig. 14. This is a dynamic reach test; you start by standing on one leg at the centre and reach out with the other leg as far as possible along each of the indicated lines (Fig. 15). Your weight should remain on your stance leg, which can bend as much as you like but the foot needs to remain flat on the floor. The 'reach' leg can brush the floor but should not be weight-bearing; by pushing a pencil or getting someone else to make a mark, record in centimetres how far you reach along each line. Repeat on the other leg and repeat 2 or 3 times on each leg.

You can examine your results in two ways. Firstly, the difference reached between the right and left legs – this can either be the sum total or the average distance reached of the 8 directions. There shouldn't be more than a 10 per cent difference between the sides. The second way is to calculate each distance reached as a percentage of your leg length. The percentage will range anywhere between 60–120 per cent depending on the direction – the anterolateral, anterior and anteromedial often have the lower scores. Again, you should look for differences above 10 per cent between the legs for areas to work on. The average percentage distance reached for all the directions for each leg should be over 100 per cent.

Inverted Y

This test has been developed from the Star Excursion Test and is a truncated version. Research on athletes has shown that using 3 directions were the best at indicating injury risk, but this link hasn't been researched on dancers. Instead of carrying out the 8 directions of the Star Excursion Test, the Inverted Y test only uses the anterior, posteromedial and posterolateral (Fig. 15) using the same technique described above.

The analysis is similar to the Star Excursion Test in that you should look for bilateral differences and the average percentage reached should be greater than 100 per cent.

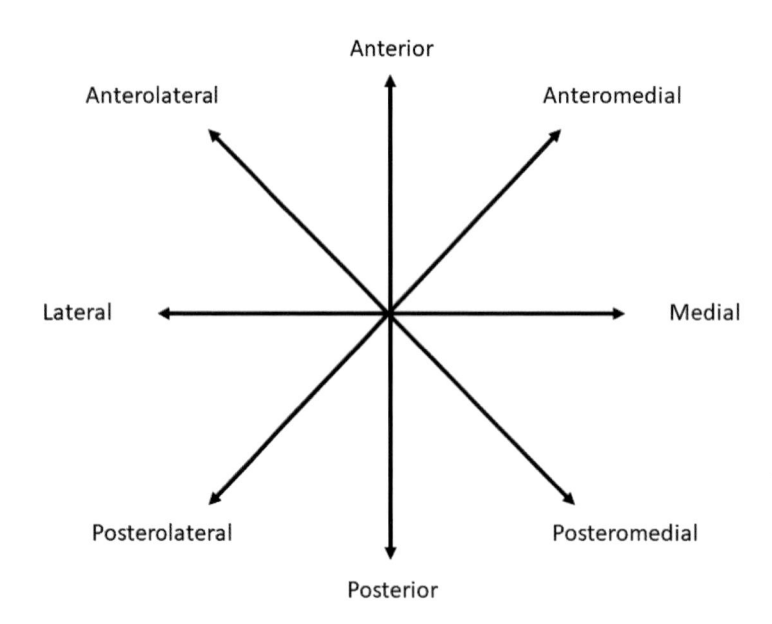

Fig. 14 Layout of the Star Excursion Test.

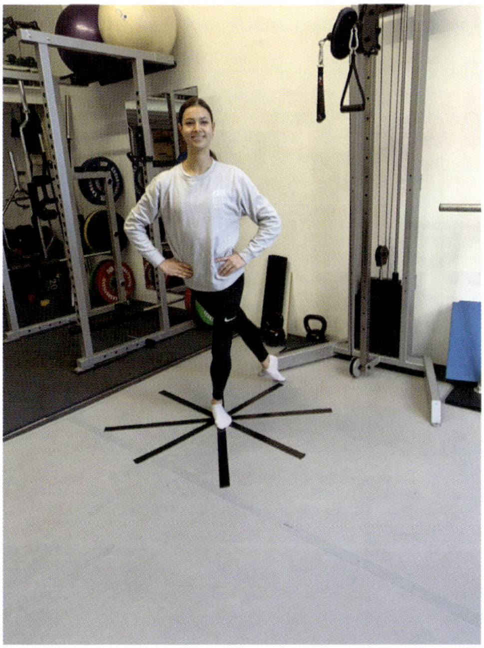

SCREENING AND PROGRAMME DESIGN

of ways to test these capacities, aerobic and anaerobic, depending on the facilities and equipment available to you. In the two dance specific tests, heart rate and Rate of Perceived Exertion (RPE, Chapter 2) are recorded at the end of each stage and as you get fitter, your heart rate and RPE will decrease. The other two tests are more simplistic and less dance specific but are just as useful to measure change. It is important to really push yourself to the maximum in these tests as otherwise you won't be able to see the improvements you've made.

Dance aerobic fitness test (DAFT)

This is a multi-stage test that starts easily and gradually gets harder with each stage. Stage 3 has the equivalent aerobic demand of a dance class and stage 5 approximately that of a dance performance.[53] Each stage is around 4 minutes long and is based around a 16-beat sequence, with intensity being increased by either increasing the tempo, the movements or the inclusion of additional movements.

Fig. 15 Participant carrying out the Star Excursion Test.

High-intensity dance performance test

As the name suggests this is a high-intensity test that takes the format of intermittent exercise. The single stage is repeated 4 times and between each attempt you are allowed

Cardiorespiratory fitness

This is one of the most important tests and is important to monitor regularly as it is fundamental to all movement. There are a number

Stage	Tempo	Movement
1	68	5 steps, lunge and recover. 4 sets of 2 pliés with 90° turn between each set.
2	78	5 steps, lunge and recover. 3 spring hops in a circle. 4 sets of 2 pliés with 90° turn between each set, arms moving between first and second position.
3	78	5 steps, lunge and recover. 3 spring hops in a circle include arm movements. 4 sets of hop plié with 90° turn between each set, arms moving between first and second position.
4	94	5 steps, lunge and recover. 3 spring hops in a circle include arm movements. 4 sets of hop, hop with 90° turn between each set, arms moving between first and second position.
5	108	5 springs, lunge and recover. 3 spring hops in a circle include arm movements. 4 sets of hop, hop with 90° turn between each set, arms moving between first and second position.

Table 5 DAFT stage descriptions.

SCREENING AND PROGRAMME DESIGN

Excellent	Completing all 5 stages with a heart rate in the last stage at 80% of your age-related maximum.
Good	Complete all 5 stages without your technique being compromised.
Average	Complete all 5 stages with compromised technique or stage 4 without your technique being compromised.
Poor	Stage 4 and below.

Table 6 What can be considered a good DAFT score?

Time	Tempo	Movement
1 min	106	4 sets of 2 jumps with 90° jump turn between each set, arms moving between first and fifth position; 2 springs forwards, roll to floor touching the back, 2 steps out into a lunge with a 180° turn to face direction you've come from; big 2-footed jump forwards with arms, mini-handstand, run backwards, star steps. Start phrase on left.
2 min		Recovery.
1 min	106	Repeat first stage but starting on right.

Table 7 High intensity dance performance test description.

Excellent	Completing all 4 stages with a heart rate in the last stage at 80% of your age-related maximum and an RPE 8/10.
Good	Complete all 4 stages without your technique being compromised.
Average	Complete all 4 stages with compromised technique or 3 stages without your technique being compromised.
Poor	Less than 3 stages.

Table 8 What can be considered a good high-intensity DAFT score?

a 2-minute recovery.[53] As you become fitter the number of repetitions you complete will increase, and heart rate and RPE decrease.

12-minute run test (Cooper's test)

This is an extremely simple test as you just need to measure the distance you can travel in 12 minutes. Notice the use of 'travel'(!) as you can run or walk (or have a rest) during this 12-minute period. With new technology, watches or phones, this is easy to do; a watch would also allow heart rate to be measured and even if you didn't cover more distance, covering the same distance at a lower heart rate indicates an improvement in cardiorespiratory fitness.

5–10–5 run test

To perform well at this test, you need to be able to change direction quickly which is a skill more developed in soccer, etc. than dance. You will need to set out the 'course': three marks 5 metres apart. For the test, you start in the middle, sprint to the far mark, back to the farthest mark and back to the middle, that is one repetition (Fig. 16); you start a new repetition

SCREENING AND PROGRAMME DESIGN

	Males	**Females**
Excellent	Over 2800 metres	Over 2700 metres
Good	2400–2800 metres	2200–2700 metres
Average	2200–2399 metres	1800–2199 metres
Poor	1600–2199 metres	1500–1799 metres

Table 9 What can be considered a good 12-min run score?

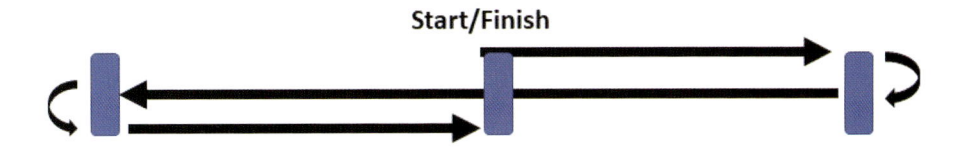

Fig. 16 5–10–5 test.

every 30 seconds. You do as many repetitions as possible before either you don't finish within 30 seconds or you keel over.

There are no norms for dancers for this test and the best way to monitor progress is repeating the test and beating your previous number of repetitions.

	Repetitions
Excellent	Over 17
Good	13–17
Average	10–12
Poor	Less than 10

Table 10 Norms for 5–10–5 test.

Flexibility

This might seem a slightly unusual parameter to measure in dancers, but the focus should be on bilateral differences in range of movement or the differences between active and passive ranges if it is possible to measure.

Beighton scoring system
This measures joint hypermobility across 5 joints on a 9-point scale: the little finger of both hands, base of both thumbs, both elbows and knees, and the spine. There is a tendency for dancers to score highly on this scale, particularly in the lower extremity. The scores of the knee and elbow are important from a safety perspective when lifting.

If you score highly on the Beighton system it could be that you are hyperflexible and not hypermobile. A simple skin pull test on the underneath of the forearm (hairless part) will indicate if you are hypermobile: if you can pull the skin away more than 1.5cm this indicates hypermobility.

If you are either hypermobile or hyperflexible, particularly in the elbows and knees, then care needs to be taken when exercising. Loaded exercises that require the limbs to be extended, such as a squat or press, need to be carried out in a controlled manner to prevent over-extension. There are enough gruesome videos online that show the results of uncontrolled movement to highlight the necessity for care.

SCREENING AND PROGRAMME DESIGN

Joint	Test	Score
Little finger	Place your palm on a flat surface and fingers out straight, with your other hand can you bend the little finger up to beyond 90 degrees?	1 point for beyond 90 degrees 1 point for each side
Thumb	With your arm out straight, the palm facing down, bend your wrist downward and gently push your thumb back to see if it can touch the forearm.	1 point for touching the forearm 1 point for each side
Elbow	Stretch your arm out to the side so your upper arm is parallel to the floor, with your palms facing up. See if your elbow extends beyond 10 degrees so your hand is lower than your elbow.	1 point for extended elbow beyond 10 degrees 1 point for each side
Knees	While standing, straighten your legs and see if your knees go beyond straight so that the lower part of the legs extend forward more than 10 degrees.	1 point for extended knee beyond 10 degrees 1 point for each side
Spine	Standing up with your legs straight, bend forward and put your hands flat on the floor.	1 point

Table 11 Beighton scoring system.

Modified Thomas test

Lie on your back on the edge of a suitable table so that your legs are hanging free. Grab one knee and pull it back to your chest with the other leg still hanging down. The back must remain flat and in contact with the table throughout. A negative test (good test) is when your back remains on the table, the grabbed knee bends more than 90 degrees and the thigh of the dangling leg remains relatively horizontal.

If there is pain in the flexed hip, there could be tightness in the psoas muscles. If your dangling knee rises up, then there is possible tightness in the quadriceps and rectus femoris. If the same leg abducts then this indicates possible tightness in the tensor fasciae latae; if the tibia rotates laterally then there is tightness in the biceps femoris.

Functional hip and hamstring flexibility

These tests resemble movements carried out in the majority of theatrical dance genres, but the principle can be applied to any joint. If you film yourself doing the test you can use free online software such as Kinovea to measure your range of movement. The first part of the test is to measure passive range of movement, i.e. to move a limb as far as it can be moved in a specific plane of motion by an external force. In reality this means how far someone else can lift your leg; you can do it using a towel or your arms (Fig. 17a), but the leg being tested needs to be totally relaxed. The second part of the test measures active range of movement: you carry out the same movement but using the muscles of your leg to move it; the movement should be controlled so it should be a développé rather than a grande battement (Fig. 17b). By carrying out the test in centre, it also challenges the support structures/anatomy involved with the movement, particularly your support leg, pelvis/hips and core stability. The test can then be repeated devant and derrière.

Analysis follows the 10-degree rule; there should only be a 10-degree difference between active and passive range of movements on one side and a 10-degree difference between left and right sides. There are some norms available to compare yourself to (Table 12) but currently there is a propensity for excessive ranges of

SCREENING AND PROGRAMME DESIGN

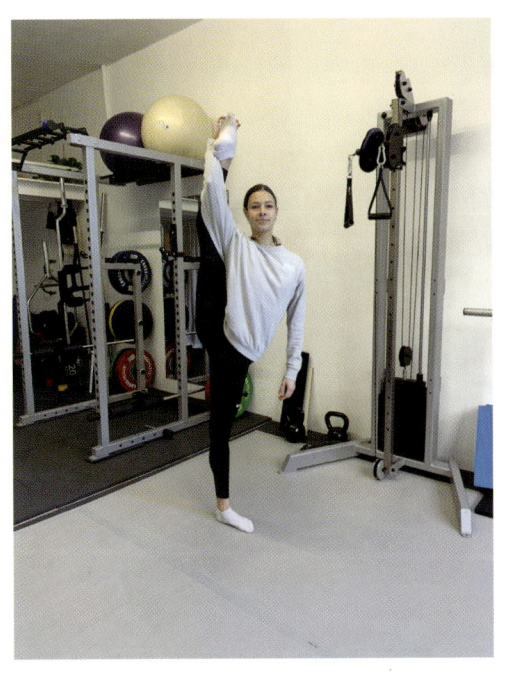

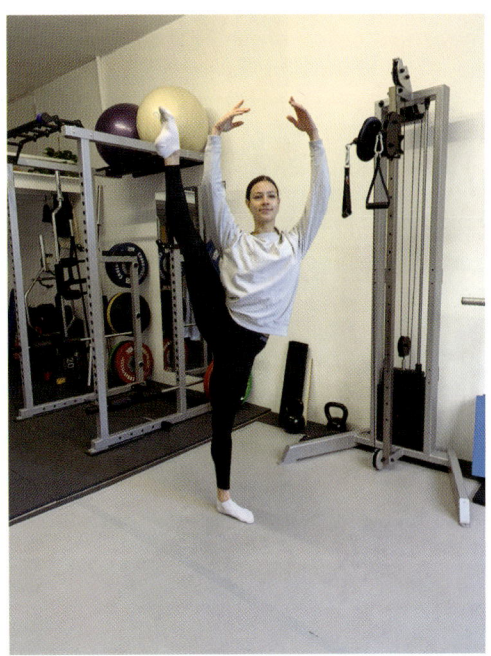

Fig. 17 a and b Passive and active hip range of movement.

Joint	Ballet	Modern	General population
Hip and hamstring flexion (passive)	Adolescent 136–1500 Professional 1200	Pre-Professional 1170	Adolescent 42–1390 Adults 48–1220
Hip and hamstring flexion (active)		University 91–1170	Adults 870
Hip and hamstring extension (passive)	Adolescent 19–320	Pre-professional 290 University 18–290	Adolescent 10–240 Adult 14–160
Hip and hamstring extension (active)	Professional 420		
Hip and hamstring flexion side (passive)	Recreational 1480 Pre-professional 127–1540 Professional (m) 125–1640 Professional (f) 175–1800	Adolescent 132–1,430 Pre-professional 116–1260 Professional 1270	
Hip and hamstring flexion side (active)	Recreational 1130 Pre-professional 95–1180 Professional (m) 195–1260 Professional (f) 145–1500	Adolescent 106–1200 Pre-professional 730 Professional 740	

Table 12 Normative hip range of movement between different genres.

SCREENING AND PROGRAMME DESIGN

movement mainly driven by social media and some choreographers. If you push yourself past your anatomical limitations, you increase the short-term risk of injury and the long-term risk of degenerative joint disease.

Lying overhead reach

This test measures the flexibility of your shoulders and lats (latissimus dorsi) muscles. This is to assess your ability to carry out specific strength exercises but is also important when lifting a partner above your head. Lie on your back with your knees bent to 90 degrees and feet flat on the floor; the length of your back should be touching the floor. Start with your arms reaching to the ceiling shoulder-width apart, but keeping the shoulders touching the floor, and slowly rotate the arms backwards above your head keeping them straight (Fig. 18).

Shoulder internal and external rotation

This is also known as the (Apley) back scratch test. Standing up raise your right arm straight up over your head and bend your right elbow. Let your right palm rest on the back of your neck with your fingers pointing down toward your feet. With your left hand, reach behind your back and rest the back of your hand on your spine with your palm facing away from your body. Try to slide your hands as close together as possible. Repeat on the other side.

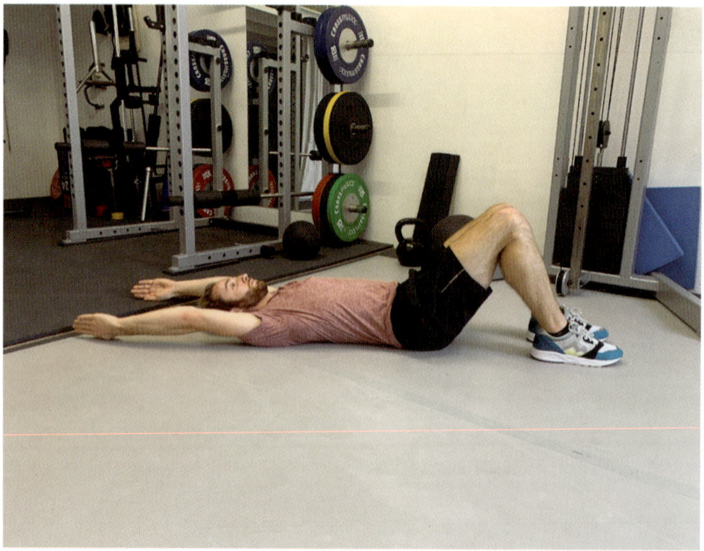

Fig. 18 Lying overhead reach test.

	Description
Excellent	Arms flat on the floor with the whole of back still in contact with the floor.
Good	Arms flat on the floor with the lower back slightly lifted.
Average	Arms reach your ears but not the floor and the whole of back still in contact with the floor.
Poor	Arms bend and remain in front of the face.

Table 13 Lying overhead reach test scoring.

SCREENING AND PROGRAMME DESIGN

	Description
Excellent	Fingers overlap
Good	Fingers touch
Average	Fingers less than 5cm apart
Poor	Fingers more than 5cm apart

Table 14 Shoulder internal and external rotation scoring.

Strength testing

Testing muscle strength is a very useful tool in that it helps monitor progress and helps set training resistance for exercise programmes. The aim is to lift or push as much weight as possible and this requires a high level of technical ability if you are to avoid injury. Therefore, these tests are not really applicable or safe for beginners. The best tests to use, though not necessarily all of them, are the squat, the deadlift, the bench press and shoulder press. Rather than attempt a 1-repetition max(imum), the maximum amount you can lift once, using a 3- or 5-repetition max is a safer option.

The squat

The squat measures lower limb strength and core strength to an extent. The depth of the squat doesn't need to be maximal, bottom to heels, but the thighs should at least be parallel to the floor at the bottom of the squat. Using a leg press or a squat using a Smith machine are safer options, but they don't engage the whole body in the same manner as a squat. There are no specific comparative data for dancers or whether strength beyond a specific level improves dance performance or injury risk than a lower strength index. Strength is often measured in body weights (BWs), amount lifted divided by your body weight, and possible indices can be found in Table 11.

The deadlift

This is a whole-body test and challenges the legs, back, core, shoulders, arms and hand grip. It is potentially safer than a squat as it is easier to release the weight. Your arms and back should remain straight and drive upwards with the hips but don't hyperextend the back at the top of the movement.

Bench and shoulder press

Ideally both these tests should be done with a free bar, but you can use a machine or Smith machine to achieve a similar effect. In chest press, the handgrip should be such that when the bar touches the chest, the elbows should be at 90°; a slightly narrower hand position is needed for the shoulder press. For both presses, you should avoid 'bouncing' the bar on your body but stop a couple of centimetres before.

Muscle power

There are two main tests that measure power: the vertical jump for the lower body and a medicine ball push for the upper body. The movements need to be fast, and you need to try to jump/push as far as you can, which is often contrary to what you do in dance.

	Squat	**Deadlift**	**Bench press**	**Shoulder press**
Excellent	2 BWs	2 BWs	1.2 BWs	1 BWs
Good	1.5 BWs	1.5 BWs	1 BW	0.7 BWs
Average	1 BW	1 BW	0.8 BWs	0.5 BWs
Poor	0.75 BWs	0.75 BWs	0.5 BWs	0.3 BWs

Table 15 Strength test indices.

SCREENING AND PROGRAMME DESIGN

Vertical jump

There are a number of types of equipment that can be used to measure jump height, these mainly measure time in the air and from this they calculate how high you've jumped. The protocol described here is more basic and requires no equipment beyond a measuring tape. Stand next to a wall with your nearest arm stretched as high as possible and mark the wall (chalk or damp fingers). Step slightly away, stand in first position and do a fast plié before jumping as high as possible. At the top of the jump slap the wall again (Fig. 19). Measure the difference between the two and this is your vertical jump height.

Medicine ball push

Sit on the floor with your back to the wall; start with the ball held straight out in front of you with straight arms before bringing the ball quickly back to the chest before pushing it away as fast as possible remembering to let go! Measure where the ball lands from the wall. There aren't any norms for dancers, but you can measure improvement by retesting after a period of training.

	Vertical jump	
	Male	Female
Excellent	60cm	40cm
Good	50cm	35cm
Average	40cm	30cm
Poor	30cm	20cm

Table 16 Vertical jump test indices.

Muscle endurance

These types of tests are easy to do, require minimal equipment, and are either timed or based on the number of repetitions performed. Most of these exercises focus on a specific group of muscles and test your ability to 'push through' localized 'pain'. As with most of the tests mentioned it is important to maintain form/technique and to stop the test when it goes; there is no point in carrying on timing a plank when you start to look like a banana.

Core endurance tests

There are a range of tests available from isometric hold tests, such as the plank and its variants, to dynamic curl tests. There is no gold standard so maybe doing two or three might give you a better idea of your capabilities, but make sure you rest in between!

Plank tests

These are the standard isometric hold tests that can be carried out in a number of different positions depending on your ability. The most basic version is the toe and elbows position (Fig. 20), with the body, legs and neck all maintaining a straight line, toes together and elbows directly under the shoulders. More advanced versions can include a side plank with one foot on top of

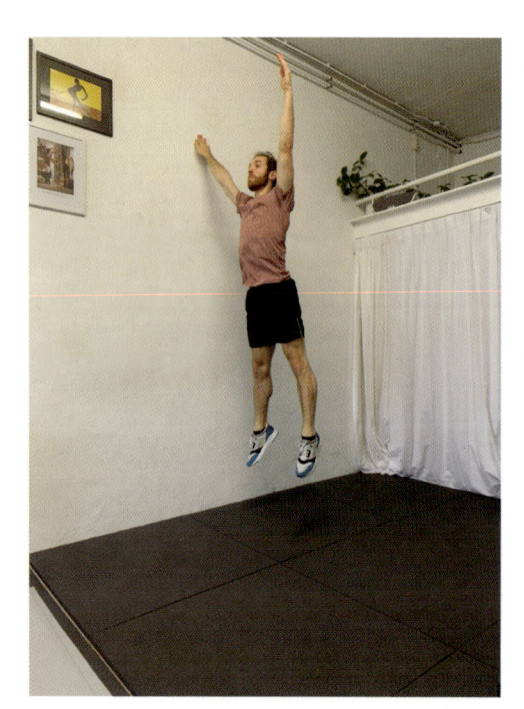

Fig. 19 Slapping the wall at the top of the jump.

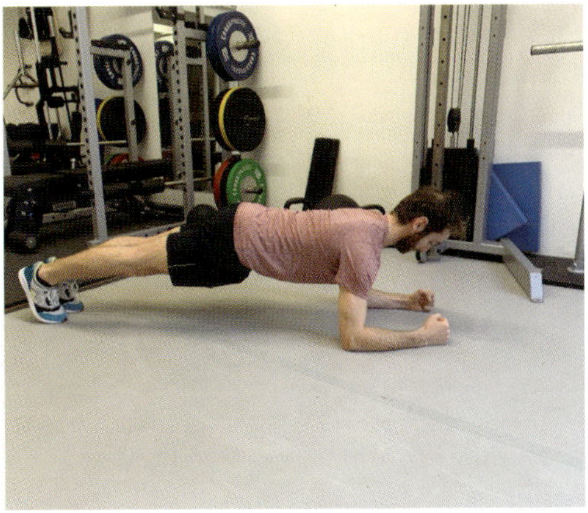

SCREENING AND PROGRAMME DESIGN

Fig. 20 Plank test position.

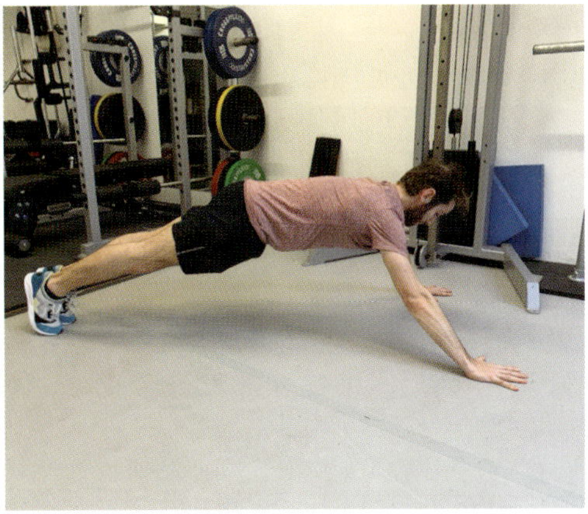

Fig. 21 Advanced plank test position.

the other and supporting elbow again directly under the shoulder; on your hand(s), with arms straight, rather than your elbows; and lastly doing the plank with your arms in front of your shoulders. To start the latter version, start lying on the floor facedown and arms out to the side at 90 degrees to the body, bend your elbows to 90 degrees, so your hands come 'above' your head, palms touching the floor. From this position push up into the plank position until your arms are straight; during the push-up phase your body and legs should remain straight (Fig. 21). This version will not only challenge your core but also your shoulder complex as well.

Scoring these tests is more of a cut off as there is little evidence that doing long periods is more beneficial. A reasonable average score is holding the position for 2 minutes and a good score is holding it for 4 minutes.

Biering Sorenson back extension test

This is the opposite test of the plank and challenges the lower back/posterior chain. If you don't have a Roman Chair, you can use a plinth or table. You need to lie with the top half of your body off the edge of the table, with the edge of the table/plinth/support across your iliac crest; obviously you need to have your legs fixed somehow either with straps or a person (Fig. 22). You need to then maintain the upper body in a horizontal position with your arms crossed over your chest. It is a timed test with the test stopping at 4 minutes or when you can no longer maintain the position.

Sit-up test and press-up test

Both of these tests follow the beat of a metronome and you carry out the continuous movement until you either can't keep up with the beat or your form goes. The cadence for both tests is forty beats per minute, up on first beat and down on second so that you complete twenty sit-ups or press-ups in a minute. Comparative scores can be found in Table 17.

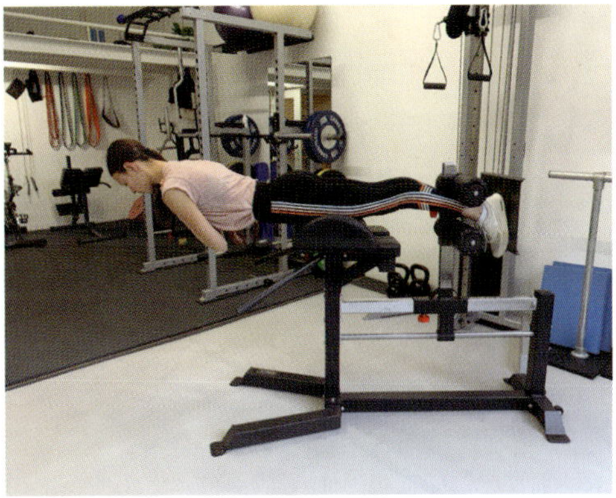

Fig. 22 Biering Sorenson back extension test.

SCREENING AND PROGRAMME DESIGN

Sit-up test: You start lying on the floor with your knees bent, feet flat on the floor, legs slightly apart, arms straight and parallel to the trunk with palms of the hands resting on the mat and the head is in contact with the mat. There should be 12cm between the tips of your fingers and the back of your heels. The feet cannot be held or rested against an object. Keeping heels in contact with the mat, you curl up slowly, sliding your fingers along the mat until you touch the back of your heels and then curl back down until your head touches the mat, that is one repetition. You should try to keep a smooth even movement on the way up and down.

Press-up test: You can do this test with either a narrow or wide hand position. The narrow position is with your hands directly under your shoulders and when you go down your arms remain close to the body; this puts a greater emphasis on your triceps than your chest. For the wide position, lie face down on the mat with your arms stretched out wide either side of you like a 'T'; place your hands where your elbows are, fingers facing forward. Start the test with your hands and toes touching the floor (knees if need be), your body and legs are in a straight line and feet slightly apart. Lower yourself down until your elbows are bent to 90 degrees (this usually corresponds to your arm being parallel to the floor) before pushing back up until your arms are fully extended. It is important that your body and legs remain in a straight line throughout the test.

Pull-up and modified pull-up test

These exercises test the opposite muscle from the press-up test. There are two versions, the full pull-up test and a modified version that will depend on your strength and equipment. The first requires a bar high enough off the ground that when you are hanging on it with fully extended arms your feet aren't touching the ground; for the modified pull-up the bar needs to be waist height. You see how many repetitions you can complete without a rest or cheating.

Pull-up: Hang from the bar with either an overhand or underhand grip and hands shoulder-width apart. Pull yourself up so that your chin touches the bar before lowering yourself back down so your arms are fully extended. The feet shouldn't touch the ground at all, and you shouldn't swing the body or legs to help getting up.

Modified test: Position yourself with your shoulders directly below the horizontal bar, using an overhand grip place your hands slightly wider than shoulder-width apart. Lift your hips so your body and legs are straight and just your heels are touching the ground when your arms are fully extended. Pull-up so your chest comes to 10cm from the bar, or your chin goes above the bar; keeping your body and legs straight return to the start position with your arms fully extended.

Single-leg calf raises

This test has gained popularity recently after the Australian Ballet demonstrated a link

	Sit-ups	Press-ups		
		Males	Females	Females (modified)
Excellent	180+	56+	30+	37+
Good	110–180	40–56	17–29	25–37
Average	64–109	19–39	9–16	12–24
Poor	below 64	Below 19	Below 9	Below 12

Table 17 Sit-up and press-up test indices.

SCREENING AND PROGRAMME DESIGN

	Pull-ups		Modified pull-ups
	Males	Females	
Excellent	14+	10+	14+
Good	11–14	5–9	11–14
Average	8–10	1–4	8–10
Poor	1		1

Table 18 Sit-up and press-up test indices.

	Number of repetitions per leg
Excellent	50+
Good	35–50
Average	20–34
Poor	Below 20

Table 19 Single-leg calf raise indices.

between poor calf endurance and injury. The test is easy to carry out: stand facing a wall (approximately 30cm away) and lightly place both hands at shoulder height, they are there solely for balance. Bend one leg slightly so it isn't touching the floor or the other leg. Keeping the test leg straight, push up through your 1st–3rd toes and not the outside of your foot until your reach full height, get someone to hold a ruler above your head at this height so you can touch it for each complete repetition. A metronome is set at 60 beats a minute, so up on one down on two. During the test avoid lifting your hip or bending and straightening your leg to get a bit of momentum. Do as many repetitions as you can before either the height of the raise is lost (head no longer touching the ruler), you start wobbling on the ascent or you can no longer keep up with the metronome. Repeat on the other leg, and there shouldn't be more than a 10 per cent difference between sides.

Functional movement screening

These types of screens are slightly more subjective but examine a complex movement that often incorporates the whole body or at least 3–4 major joints. If you are self-analysing, then it is a good idea to film yourself doing the activity. In all the below tests you should be looking for smooth, controlled movement that utilizes the full range of movement. When there are imbalances, these manifest themselves as compensatory or restricted movement such as arm wafting, knee wobble, movement off a straight line. Below we will describe the tests and also highlight possible causes of the main compensatory movements.

Triple hop

This is a very simple test: you want to measure how far you can travel with three continuous hops on one leg without the other touching

Poor distance or a big difference between legs	This can be due to two main things: firstly, a lack of power in the leg, and secondly a lack of control during landing and push-off.
You veer off in one direction	This is mainly due to a lack of control during the landing and push-off phases due to poor alignment on the leg kinetic chain. Look at the ankle, knee and hip joint to see what is happening – they should be 'stacked' one on top of the other. Also look at the direction the knee is 'pointing' in – is it pointing over the toes or off to one side?
You lose balance and the other foot touches the floor	See above.

Table 20 Triple hop: things to look for.

SCREENING AND PROGRAMME DESIGN

the ground, and then repeat on the other leg. The test is examining your ability to generate power (hop distance) and remain balanced. Good scores are over 6.5m for males and 4.7m for females. The 10 per cent rule applies here as well, in that there should be no more than a 10 per cent difference between the distances covered.

Hurdle jump onto one leg and fix landing

This is a simplified version of the triple hop test and is good to do especially if you are having landing leg alignment issues. Set a pole or band at a height of 50 per cent of your vertical jump test height, or around 15cm for females and 20cm for males. Standing approximately 30cm behind the pole, you want to do a two-footed take-off to jump over the pole and then land on one leg. On landing you want to hold that position for 3 seconds. Again, carry out on both legs.

Overhead squat

This is a whole-body test that examines the co-ordination and range of movement of the lower legs, torso and upper limbs. Start with your feet shoulder-width apart and your feet in parallel; raise your arms above your head,

Foot shuffle, arm wafting, torso bending	This is mainly due to a lack of control during the landing due to poor alignment on the leg kinetic chain. Look at the ankle, knee and hip joint to see what is happening – they should be 'stacked' one on top of the other.
Knee 'collapses' inwards	This is probably due to overactive thighs and underactive glutes.
You lose balance and the other foot touches the floor	See above.

Table 21 Hurdle jump: things to look for.

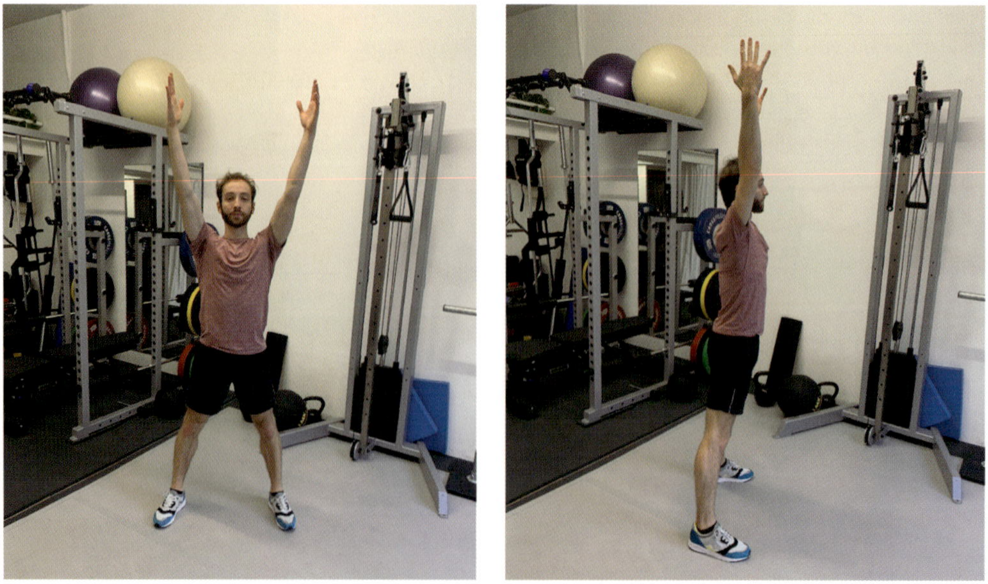

Fig. 23 a and b Start position for overhead squat.

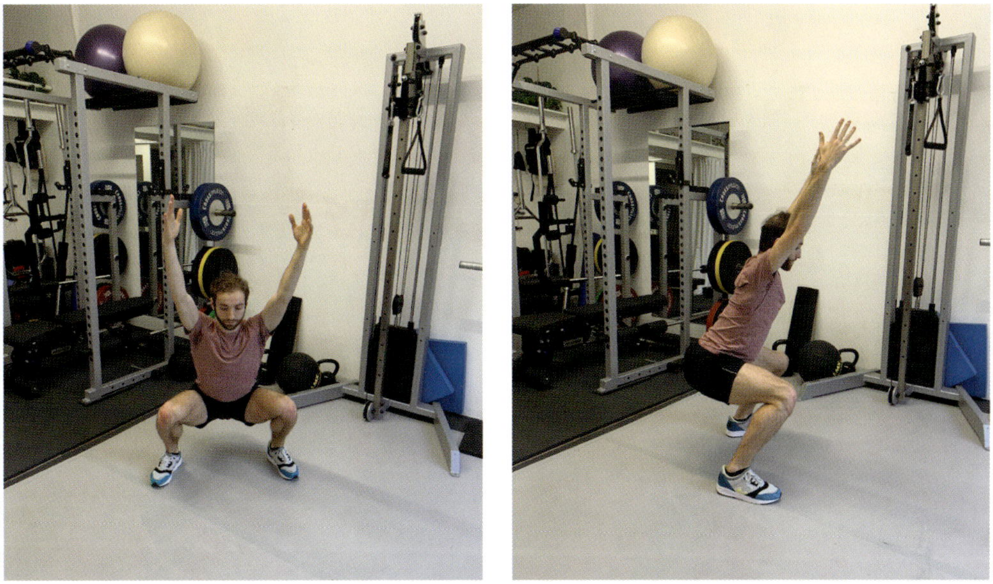

SCREENING AND PROGRAMME DESIGN

Fig. 24 a and b Bottom position for the overhead squat.

Excessive forward lean	This is probably due to overactive calf muscles, hip flexors and/or abs as well as underactive glutes, shins, and/or medial back.
Arms fall forward	This is probably due to overactive back muscles and/or chest muscles as well as underactive upper back muscles and/or rotator cuff.
Lower back arch	This is probably due to overactive hip flexors and/or back as well as underactive glutes, hamstrings and/or the intrinsic core stabilizer muscles.
Knees move inward	This is probably due to overactive thighs and underactive glutes.
Feet turn out	This is probably due to overactive calf muscles and part of your quadricep as well as underactive calf muscles, hamstrings and adductors.

Table 22 Overhead squat: things to look for.

ideally with your elbows close to your ears, palms of your hands facing each other. Your head and neck should be in line with the spine, with eyes looking forward, and your hands should be directly over your feet (Figs 23a and b). Now try to squat down, bottom to heels whilst keeping your head looking forward, your back straight and your hands still directly over your feet (Figs 24a and b). Return to the standing position, trying to maintain your arm position.

Step-up on a bench

You start by standing upright in front of a box or platform that is approximately knee height. Place one foot on top of the box, keeping your hands by your side. Now, trying to keep your body, neck and head upright, push up with the leg whose foot is on the box so you can stand on the box. The movement needs to be done in a controlled manner. Now reverse the movement by stepping down, leaving the same foot on the box, also in a controlled manner.

63

SCREENING AND PROGRAMME DESIGN

Excessive forward lean	This is probably due to overactive calf muscles, hip flexors and/or abs as well as underactive glutes, shins, and/or medial back.
Knees move inward	This is probably due to overactive thighs and underactive glutes.
Feet turn out	This is probably due to overactive calf muscles and part of your quadricep as well as underactive calf muscles, hamstrings and adductors.

Table 23 Step-up test: things to look for.

Physiotherapy screen

It is often a good idea to have a yearly screen by a physiotherapist, irrespective of whether you have been injured or not. They will be able to test your muscles and joints to look for imbalances or limitations and develop an exercise programme to provide balance. It is a good idea to find a physio with dance or at least sport medicine experience, as they will have a better understanding of what is normal for your activity.

Screening review

A good way to start is to rank all the components you screened from best to worst. The top three components are the things you are excellent at and should be proud of; it is the bottom three things that need your attention. The idea is to develop a programme that will make these bottom components as good as your top three components without losing your abilities in the components you are good at. This requires you to split the components again into 'components to work on' and 'components to maintain'. You now know what to focus on when designing your programme.

PROGRAMME DESIGN

There are no right or wrong ways of developing the ideal programme for you. You will need to experiment to see how you respond to different sessions and how they affect your dancing. To get you started or to give a variation on what you are currently doing, we have provided six 'ready-made' programmes for you to do: two each for beginners, intermediate and advanced (*see* Chapter 10).

Things to think about

Priorities

We have provided a number of ways of determining what you need to do, whether it is via needs analysis, screening or what research has suggested are areas of weakness for dancers. The most important thing when designing your own programme is to keep it simple. It is very easy to become overwhelmed with all the different things you could or should do. It is good to split the different components into two categories: components you are good at, and components that need working on. The aim over time is to gradually move all the components into the 'good at' category; this won't be achieved in a couple of months but over a number of years.

Quality, not quantity

Training sessions don't need to take a long time, as it is often the social aspects (chatting) that elongate sessions; a session can be just 20 minutes long and still achieve the desired effect. Get in, train focused, get out.

Fitting it all in

When designing your programme, it is very important to do it in relation to what you are doing during your dance training. The supplemental training is there to support your dancing, not compromise it! You don't have to do all your training together on the same day if you have a very busy schedule, but you can spread it out across the week. On busy days you might be able to just do one 20-minute session but on quieter days 2–4 sessions.

How much is enough?
Components to work on will require two sessions a week, whilst those in maintenance need to be trained maybe just once a week or fortnight. For instance, if 'jump height' is in maintenance mode and during your dance training you are doing a lot of jumps during class and/or rehearsal, then a once-a-fortnight plyometric session would be enough to maintain this component. But if your current dance training doesn't include jumps then a once-a-week session would be needed.

Exercise order
Should you do CV training before resistance training? This is the normal order you find in most health clubs and is mainly down to two things: firstly, most people don't enjoy CV training and it's boring, so by doing it first, they are less likely to skip it; secondly, it does warm up the body ready for resistance training. Another common practice is to train the large muscle groups before smaller groups; this is because the smaller groups fatigue faster and would limit the ability to train the larger muscles afterwards. For you the order should be about importance: train the components that need developing the most first, whether it is resistance or CV training. The exception is for high load exercises such as plyometrics and some Olympic lifts. These shouldn't be carried out when you are fatigued, as you need to maintain alignment during these high force movements.

Training legs
As legs are an essential part of dancing, it is important that you plan your supplemental leg training carefully, especially if you are developing strength or power. Immediately after a hard strength or power training session, you will experience a drop in neuromuscular control, particularly fine motor control, for approximately 3–4 hours. Therefore trying to do anything skilful or elegant in this time period is difficult; this also applies to maintaining alignment during landings. The ability to jump could also be compromised for the next 24–36 hours as the muscle repairs itself. Therefore, planning needs to be done with care so it doesn't affect your dancing. If you have the weekend off or a couple of easy dance days then a leg session just prior to that will be ideal. It is just as important not to avoid training the legs. Dancers generally have relatively weak leg strength and research has shown increased leg strength not only increases performance factors but also protects against injury.

Training the foundation
It is important to train the foundations before moving on to the exciting, more dance-related training. Initially training your core and stabilizers before starting strength training is essential (before moving onto plyometrics, etc.). In just the same thread, you need to develop a strong aerobic foundation before starting interval or HIIT. If you skip ahead then often future training goals are affected; for instance, a poor aerobic base means that during an HIIT session the recovery between the high-intensity periods is slower and therefore affects the subsequent high-intensity period and the overall number of periods achieved. It is a similar situation for plyometric training: without prior strength training, your anatomical structures won't have the resilience to cope with the plyometric forces and recovery will take longer.

Variety is the spice of life
It is very easy to always do the same exercises when training, but it is important to vary the movement pattern we use when training a specific muscle, or group of muscles. This is because a major aspect of training is neuromuscular and if you always keep to the same movement pattern then there is reduced crossover of benefits to other movement patterns

using the same muscle. Using a monthly rotation of exercises will help prevent monotony.

Progression
One of the limitations of current dance training is that after an initial increase in training load, the demands on the body flatten out and the body starts to become more and more efficient. As we have described before, our body is an adaptive organism that responds to new challenges. The new challenge will eventually become easy and that is when you need a new stimulus, either by increasing the workload/resistance/speed or by changing the movement pattern.

Train for what you will be doing, not what you are currently doing
Suddenly realizing you need to be stronger or fitter for what you are presently doing is too late. Training adaptation takes time, so you need to plan ahead to prepare yourself for what you are about to do in three to four months' time. As your fitness base becomes greater, this specific preparation period will get shorter.

Plan rest, recovery and eating
Rest and recovery are fundamental to good training. This isn't just concerning supplemental fitness training but all of your training. Coupled with this is getting enough good quality sleep with at least an hour of deep sleep. Just as important is making sure you fuel yourself properly – eat for what you are about to do, not what you have just done. This might require planning meals and when to eat them in advance, rather than leaving it to chance and what's available at a local shop.

Missing a session
Training, whether it be dancing or fitness training, is about the accumulation of all your training and not a single session. If you have a heavy schedule, had a bad night's sleep, are stressed, etc., it is okay to miss a class or workout. It is more important to recover and feel healthy than to squeeze in the session and do it poorly. You shouldn't feel that you have to play 'catch-up' either; move on and focus on the next session.

Have FUN
All training needs to be enjoyable, though the joy might occur post session rather than during it. You should look forward to each session – whether it is a technique class, rehearsal, or fitness session – and know how the session is helping you be a better dancer.

5 PILATES FOR DANCERS

by Aline Nogueira Haas

PILATES METHOD

History

The Pilates Method (PM) was created by Joseph Pilates at the beginning of the twentieth century. Since his childhood, Pilates had always been involved with body culture, his main influences being gymnastics, boxing and strength training. Initially known as the 'art and science of Contrology', the PM was defined by Joseph Pilates as the complete coordination of body, mind and spirit.

He moved to England in around 1913–14, probably to further his interest in boxing and body conditioning, and hoping to learn more from his compatriot, Eugene Sandow, a bodybuilder and strength expert. During the First World War he was interned on the Isle of Man and here he had the opportunity to teach body conditioning and boxing and started to develop his own exercise method.

Pilates returned to Germany in 1919 and worked as a boxing coach and athlete. He also taught self-defence to police officers and worked with the physical rehabilitation of wounded soldiers in hospitals. It was in the latter environment that he dedicated more time and energy to develop his exercise method, and designed and built his first apparatus, the Foot Corrector.

In 1926, Pilates moved to New York and established his first studio on 8th Avenue. On the voyage to New York, he met Clara Zeuner, who would become his wife and work partner. While living in New York, he continued teaching, developing his exercise method and building exercise apparatus.

For many years, in the studio in New York, Joseph Pilates worked with dancers and rehabilitating and preventing injuries. George Balanchine, Ruth St Denis, Ted Shawn, Martha Graham, Hanya Holm and Jerome Robbins were among the famous dancers that worked closely with Joseph Pilates. Another important contact with dancers was at the Jacob's Pillow Festival, a renowned summer camp for dancers, coordinated and organized by Ted Shawn. Pilates taught body conditioning for dancers at the Festival from 1942 to 1943 and from 1947 to 1951.

Joseph Pilates worked with dancers for almost forty years, from the opening of his first studio in New York until his death. It is important to highlight that the first PM followers and disciples, who continued the method, were dancers, including Romana Kryzanowska,

Eve Gentry, Ron Fletcher, Kathy Grant and Carola Trier, among others. This first generation of disciples, considered the Pilates 'elders', was responsible for keeping the PM alive and passing it on, spreading the method worldwide. The PM has historically been used as supplementary training for dancers, helping them to prevent injuries, rehabilitate after injury and improve performance.

Characteristics

The PM is a physical conditioning method that combines flexibility, strength, resistance and balance training. It is a 'body and mind' method, which is the conscious control of all muscular movements of the body. It is the correct utilization and application of the leverage principles afforded by the skeletal framework of the body, a complete knowledge of the mechanism of the body, and a full understanding of the principles of equilibrium and gravity as applied to the movements of the body in motion. Movement coordination occurs through the powerhouse or core; this is the area of the body between the bottom of the ribcage and the pelvic floor, including the diaphragm, abdominals, pelvic floor, spine and hip muscles.

The purpose of the PM exercises is to work the powerhouse and the whole-body muscles. The focus is on the movements of the spine (flexion, extension, rotation, lateral flexion), connecting the torso with the upper and lower limbs, improving strength, flexibility, balance and diminishing imbalance between agonist and antagonist muscles (such as strengthening the abdominals and back muscles to balance the core muscles). There is an understanding that in the PM the torso is crucial to the correct performance of the movements (the movements radiate out from the centre to the body extremities).

The PM is a system of movement that uses a varied set of exercises, more than 500; this incorporates mat work, apparatus (such as the Reformer, Cadillac, Chairs, Barrels, Guillotine and so on), and accessories (such as toe and foot corrector, bean bag, magic circle and so on). Some mat exercises can be performed on the apparatus, with the addition of springs providing more resistance or assistance during the exercises (facilitating or making them harder). Repetitions of each exercise do not go above 5–10 repetitions in general, with the focus firmly on the quality of the execution and not the number of repetitions. A fundamental aspect of all PM movements is the movement speed, with Pilates promoting steady, controlled movements that flow.

Mat work

This is the foundation of the method; it incorporates a series of exercises that are done on the floor. On the mat, your body uses gravity as a resistance during the movements. Joseph Pilates proposed in his book a specific order in which the exercises were to be followed.

Reformer apparatus

This is a carriage with four or five springs, which moves back and forwards and was developed 'to reorganize', 'remodel' and strengthen the whole body. Once again, Joseph Pilates developed a series of exercises with a specific pre-established order to stimulate the muscles with a focus on engaging or re-engaging the correct muscles during exercises.

Other apparatus and accessories

Using other apparatus and accessories, you can develop specific skills with direction from a qualified practitioner. The selection of exercises can be tailored to the choreographic demands you are preparing for and should be largely dependent upon your individual training requirements, in order to improve motor control of fine movements through the development of a finely tuned body awareness.

PILATES FOR DANCERS

Principles

The PM has six basic principles: centring, concentration, control, precision, breath and flow, which are important for understanding the philosophy of the method and guide the way the exercises should be performed. The six principles can help you increase core strength, range of motion, overall body awareness, correct alignment and posture, leading to a better technique and performance, and possibly help prevent injuries.

Centring

This is the main focus of the PM. All work begins in the powerhouse, strengthening the powerhouse, means strengthening the muscles that support the spine and internal organs, such as abdominals, pelvic floor and hip muscles. By having a strong powerhouse, it is possible to build a stable basis in the body that helps you to perform exercises with quality and accuracy.

Concentration

All the PM exercises should be performed with concentration, using the following aspects of the mind: intuition, intelligence, imagination, memory and desire. The mind guides the body, and the attention to all parts of the body is important. The performance of the movements and/or exercises requires maximum focus and therefore shouldn't be done when tired.

Control

Movement control is when exercises originate from the powerhouse and you have total concentration. This means you are paying close attention to all the movement details, guaranteeing the correct recruitment of muscles.

Precision

All exercises have a clear structure, and a precise way to perform them. The PM works with movement quality, not with quantity. Precision reduces the risk of injuries and improves movement control. To work with precision, it is necessary to be totally concentrated and connected with the centre (powerhouse).

Breath

The PM exercises are performed with a natural breathing pattern. The breathing pattern is called lateral or intercostal breathing (breath in wide and full to the sides of the ribcage). This breathing pattern promotes the full use of the ribcage and respiratory muscles.

Flow

Rhythm is fundamental to challenge all the other principles. The flow happens in the PM in between repetitions and exercises. Flow generates movement and movement generates blood circulation.

Systems

The PM is divided into four systems: basic, intermediate, advanced and super advanced. All systems include mat work, apparatus and accessories. To change systems (one system to another), progressions and variations of the exercises are gradually introduced, challenging the exercises' angles and postures.

Basic system

This is 'the soul' of the method. The main purpose is strengthening the powerhouse and focusing on the pelvic girdle muscles to foster stabilization and change the body from the centre out to the extremities. Apparatus: mat, Reformer, Cadillac, High Chair and exercises against a wall.

Intermediate system

Gradually new exercises and variations are introduced, with more apparatus and accessories and an increased emphasis on movement quality (flow). The focus is on strengthening the powerhouse and the pelvic and shoulder girdle muscles to foster stabilization through stretching and strengthening the relative muscles.

PILATES FOR DANCERS

Advanced system
Full body activation with movements radiating from the powerhouse. Current and new exercises are designed to be more challenging and require greater control as the angles and positions of the body vary more. More emphasis is placed on the flow of the movements.

Super advanced system
Greater engagement of the full body powerhouse movements, often becoming acrobatic, through even more challenging body positions that require a lot of control. Continuation in the development of movement flow.

PILATES METHOD FOR DANCERS

With dancers' intense training schedules, the PM can be used as a supplementary training technique to improve their performance. The PM helps to build crucial physical capacities for dance performance such as good alignment, posture, flexibility and the core muscle resistance through breathing, without neglecting the artistic component. Also, it can be beneficial to dancers for all genres, allowing them to develop the necessary underlying physical capabilities.

One of the reasons the method was enthusiastically embraced by dancers was its similarity to dance, particularly due to its underlying principles as well as some of the exercises. Although the evidence is very limited for dance, the PM has been shown to improve (to moderate effect) dynamic alignment of the torso in young ballet dancers;[54] muscular strength and flexibility in dance students;[55] postural stability and abdominal strength in young female dancers;[56] flexibility, strength and pelvic alignment.[57] Despite this, research hasn't reported a benefit of Reformer-based training on jump height or pelvic alignment when dancers performed a standing jump.[58] The PM will enable good postural alignment accompanied by a balance between core strength and whole-body flexibility, thereby allowing the body to work efficiently.

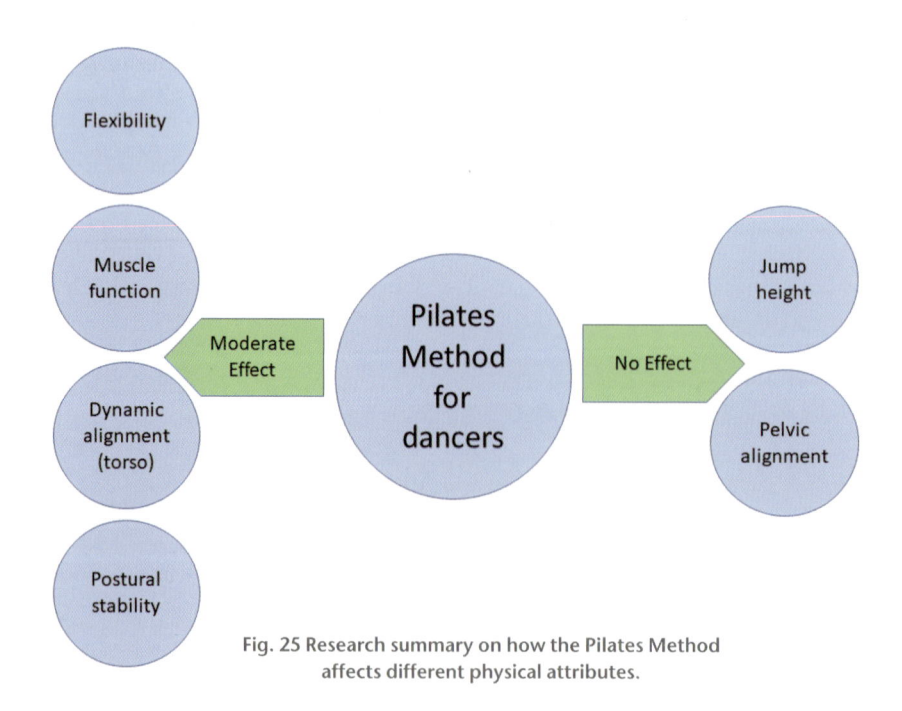

Fig. 25 Research summary on how the Pilates Method affects different physical attributes.

PILATES FOR DANCERS

PILATES METHOD BASIC MAT WORK EXERCISES

The mat work basic sequence could help you to align the body and improve posture, working core strength and whole-body flexibility. This 15- to 20-minute sequence can be added to your routine, scheduled either before or after training.

Hundred

Objectives:

- Warm-up
- Works the abdominal and core muscles
- Activates body circulation and breathing
- Increases lung capacity (breathing exercise)

Repetitions: 10 series × 10 breaths (5 inhale, 5 exhale).
Set-up position: lie on the mat with arms by your sides, reaching towards feet; curl up so the top of the back is off the floor.

Basic: legs in 'table-top' position.
Intermediate: legs at 45-degree angle.
Advanced/super advanced: legs 5cm from the mat.
Movement: pumping the arms vigorously, up and down.
Breathing pattern: inhale for 5 counts, exhale for 5 counts.

Half roll down

Objectives:

- Mobilizes and flexes the spine
- Works abdominal muscles and the core
- Works the 'C' curve in the spine

Repetitions: 5–10.
Set-up position: knees bent, legs hip-width apart, feet on the floor, hands behind the thighs, capital 'C' in the spine ('C curve').
Movement: whilst inhaling, curl the tailbone under and roll back until the arms are

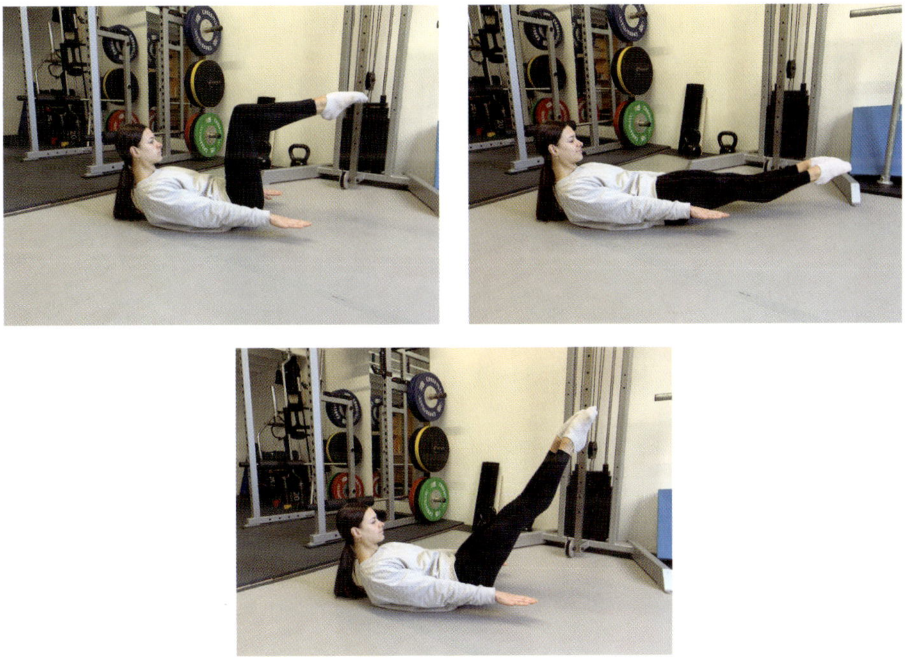

Fig. 26 Hundred set-up positions.

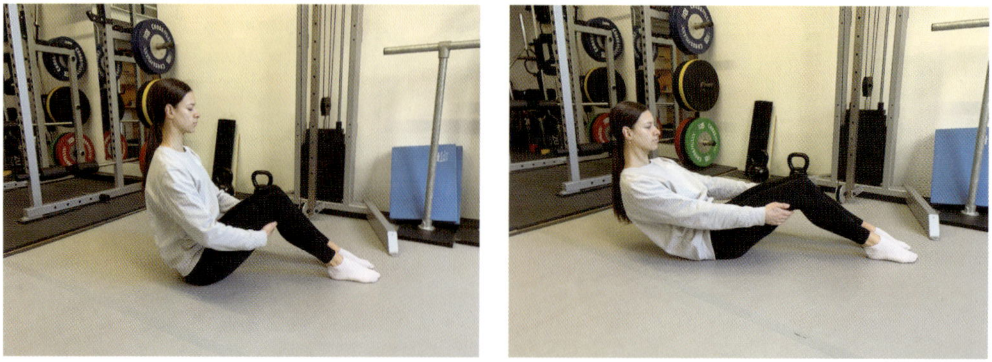

PILATES FOR DANCERS

Fig. 27 Half roll down set-up position and movement.

straight. During the exhale, roll back up to start position. Keep the 'C' curve during the movement.

Roll up
Objectives:

- Mobilizes and flexes the spine
- Works the abdominal and core muscles
- Works the 'C' curve in the spine
- Stretches the posterior (back) chain
- Increases lung capacity (breathing exercise)
- Stabilizes shoulder girdle

Repetitions: 5–10.
Set-up position: knees bent, legs together, feet flexed, arms to the ceiling.

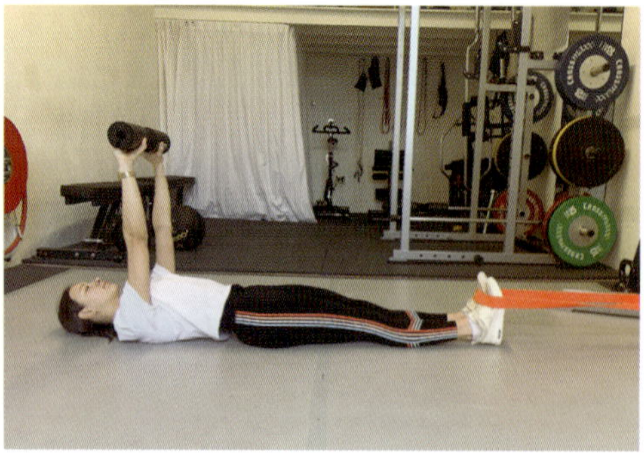

Fig. 28 Roll up.

Movement: whilst inhaling, bring the head between the arms; whilst exhaling, roll up. Inhale at the top of the movement before exhaling whilst rolling down vertebra by vertebra.

One leg circle
Objectives:

- Stabilizes the pelvic and shoulder girdles and the spine
- Develops body alignment and body control
- Stretches the posterior (back) chain
- Dissociates hip joint

Repetitions: 5 in each direction (both legs).
Set-up position: lie on the mat; arms to the side, reaching towards the feet. Extend one leg along the mat, and one leg to the ceiling.
Movement: circle the lifted leg toward the midline (moving the leg in the direction of the opposite shoulder), and then around. Reverse the direction. Repeat on the other side.

Rolling like a ball
Objectives:

- Stabilizes the pelvic and shoulder girdles
- Massages the spine and the internal organs

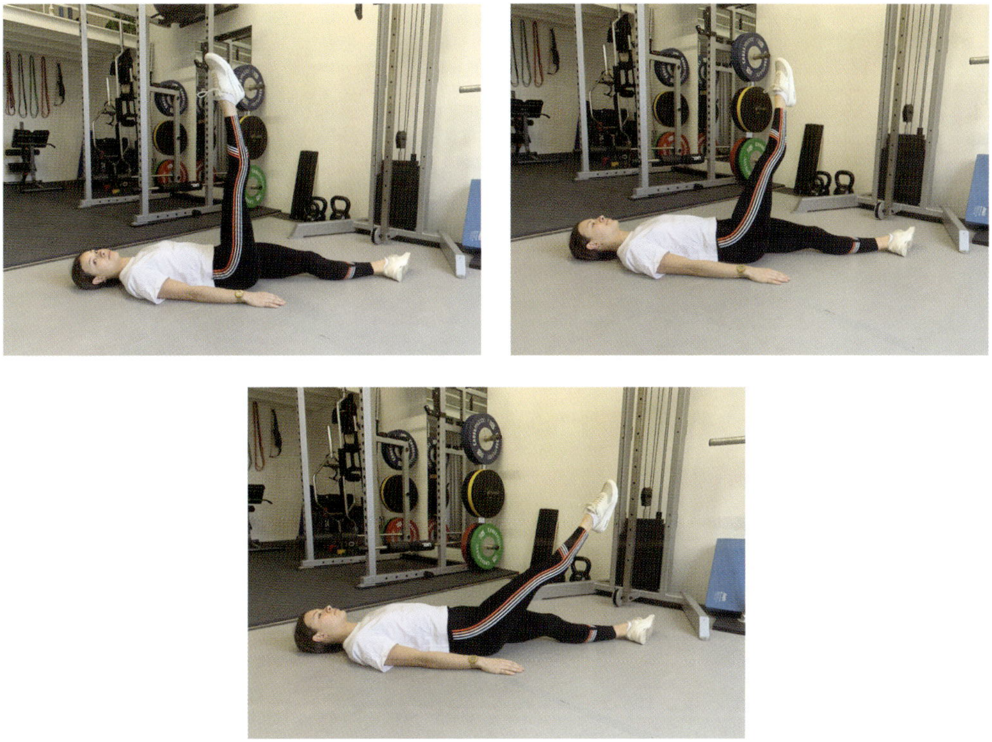

PILATES FOR DANCERS

Fig. 29 One leg circle.

- Develops balance
- Works the 'C' curve in the spine
- Works abdominal and core muscles

Repetitions: 5–10.
Set-up position: sitting up with your legs bent and together, hold onto the ankles. Round your spine into the 'C' position and tuck your chin between your knees.
Movement: as you inhale, roll backwards onto the shoulders, and as you exhale roll back to the seated position – 'rolling like a ball'.

Single leg stretch
Objectives:

- Works the abdominal and core muscles
- Stabilizes the pelvic and shoulder girdles

- Develops coordination and improves alignment
- Increases lung capacity (breathing exercise)

Repetitions: 8–10 on each leg.
Set-up position: lie on the mat with the knees pulled into the chest, curl the upper body up so the tips of the shoulder blades are just touching the mat and your eyes are looking to the belly button. Place your right hand on the right ankle and left hand on the right knee. Extend the left leg out so it is around 20cm off the mat.
Movement: whilst inhaling pull the bent knee into the chest, reaching out with the straight leg. Whilst exhaling, switch the legs and hand positions so the left leg is now tucked to the chest and the right leg is extended out, all the while keeping your upper body still and stable.

73

PILATES FOR DANCERS

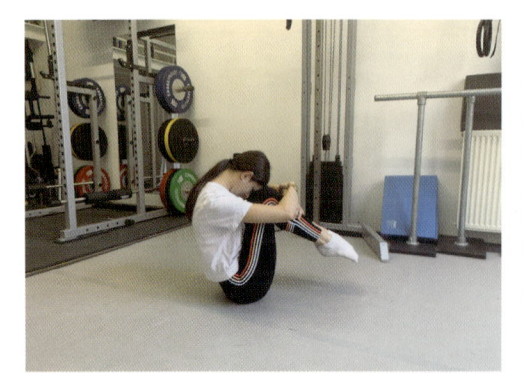

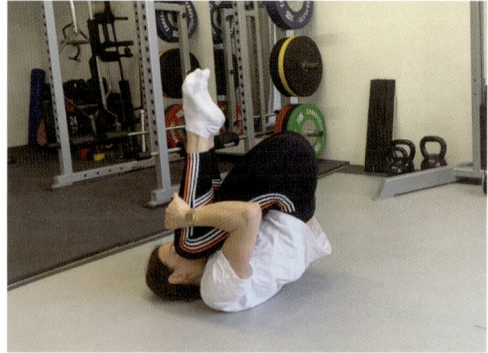

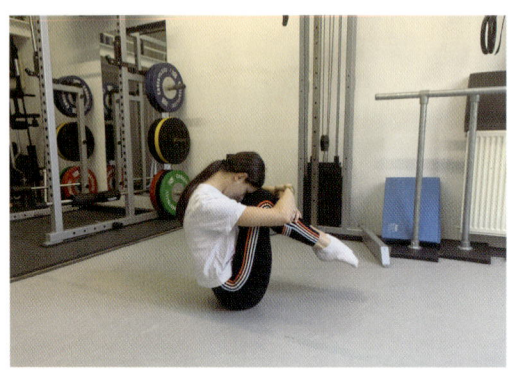

Fig. 30 Rolling like a ball.

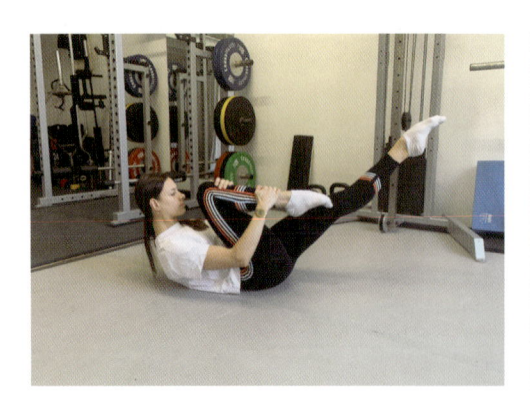

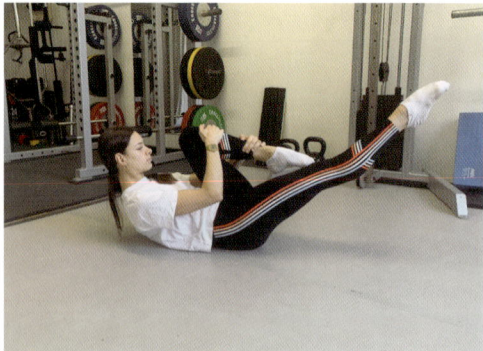

Fig. 31 Single leg stretch.

Double leg stretch
Objectives:

- Works the abdominal and core muscles
- Stabilizes the pelvic and shoulder girdles
- Develops coordination and improves alignment
- Increases lung capacity (breathing exercise)

Repetitions: 8–10.

Set-up position: lie on the mat with the knees into the chest, hands around the ankles, curl the upper body up so the tips of the shoulder

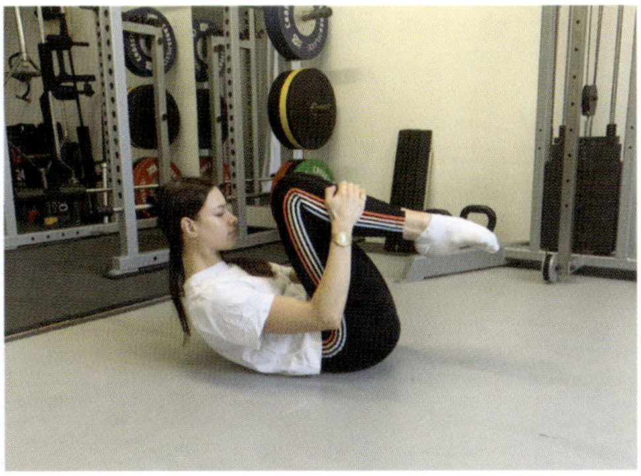

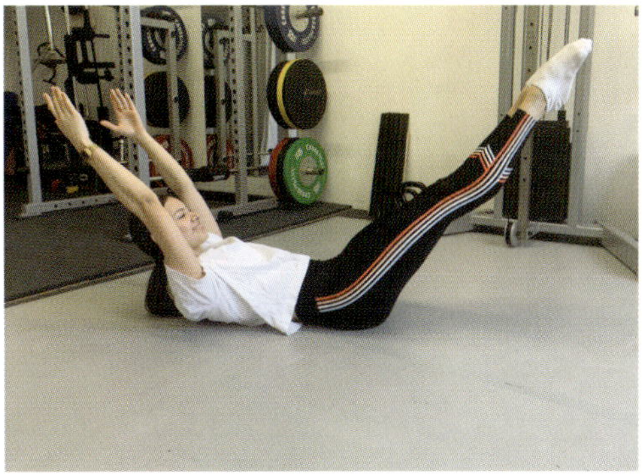

PILATES FOR DANCERS

Fig. 32 Double leg stretch.

blades are just touching the mat and your eyes are looking to the belly button.

Movement: whilst inhaling, extend your arms back (by the ears) whilst simultaneously extending the legs out, reaching opposite directions. Whilst exhaling, return to the set-up position, circling the arms and hugging the knees.

Spine stretch forward

Objectives:

- Increases lung capacity (breathing exercise)
- Stretches the posterior (back) chain
- Stabilizes the pelvic and shoulder girdles
- Stretches and mobilizes the spine muscles
- Works axial elongation in the spine

Repetitions: 5.

Set-up position: sit tall, legs extended wide, arms forward at shoulder height.

Movement: whilst inhaling, lengthen the spine; whilst exhaling bring the chin into the chest, rolling down the spine as you reach the arms forward, keeping them in line with the shoulders. Whilst inhaling gradually re-stack the spine to return to the start position.

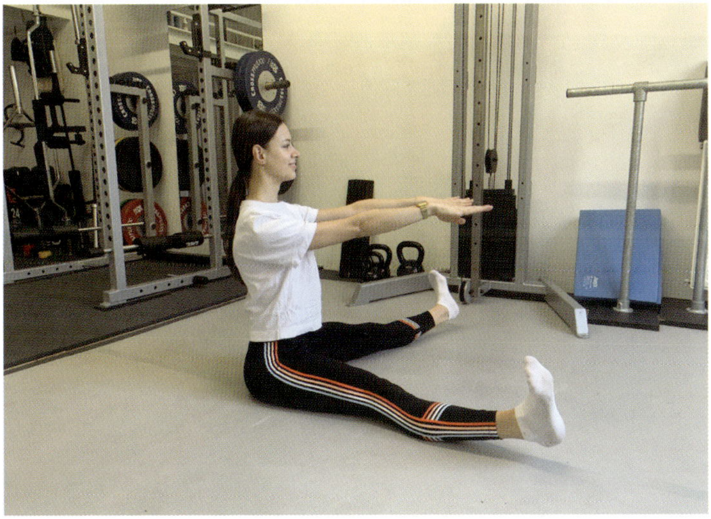

Fig. 33 Spine stretch forward.

6 CORE EXERCISES

We recognize that the exercises outlined within this chapter are not an exhaustive list and that there are many other exercises and variations. The idea is to hopefully provide you with some solid exercises, some of which might be new or forgotten.

Dead bugs

This is known as an anti-extension exercise and will help you to feel how your 'core' should be working during an exercise. This is also a great way to begin creating trunk stiffness and intra-abdominal pressure and by using the legs and arms as levers you can create more or less work for the core to do simply by shortening or lengthening them, which makes this a very scalable and easy-to-progress exercise.

1. Lie supine on the ground and raise your legs to 90 degrees. Raise your arms so that they are in line with your shoulders with your palms facing each other (Fig. 34).
2. Your lower back should very lightly be touching the ground. There mustn't be too

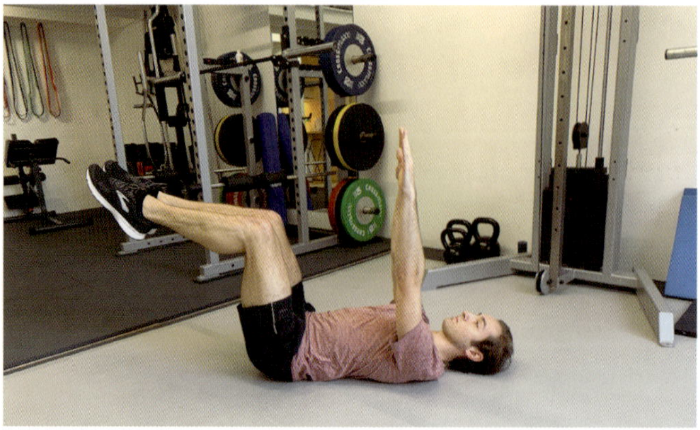

Fig. 34 Dead bug start position.

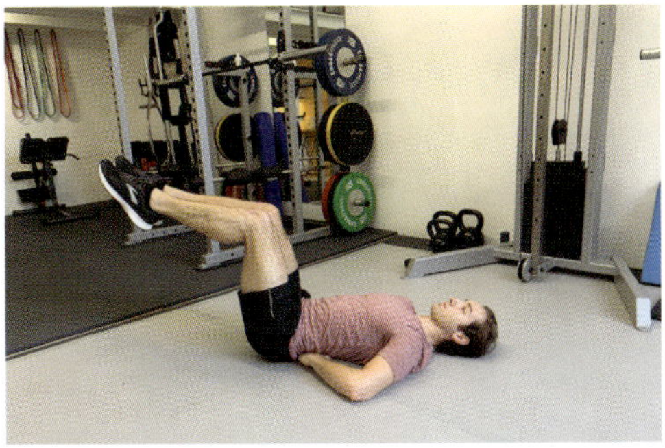

CORE EXERCISES

Fig. 35 Lower back position.

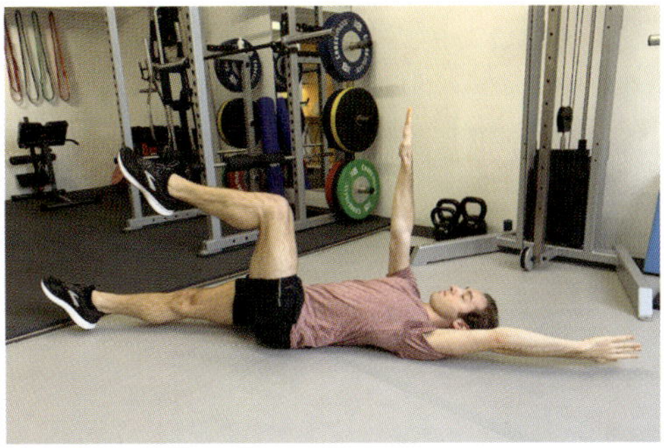

Fig. 36 Movement.

much pressure placed here. The idea is that if needed you could slide a piece of paper underneath it (Fig. 35).

3. Slowly lower one leg and the opposite arm until they reach the ground without the lower back going into extension (Fig. 36). If this happens you can regress this simply by shortening the arms or legs so that they are closer to the body or by taking out either the arms, so that only the legs are working, or the legs so that only the arms are working.

Dead bugs with resistance

1. Line up with a cable station and set the cable so that it runs parallel with the floor. Choose your selected weight which should only be heavy enough so that you can continue to breathe throughout the exercise.
2. Lie on the ground just far enough away so that when you take the ropes and put your arms in a straight line with your shoulders the weight stack lifts. Your legs should be at a 90-degree angle with your hips and your lower back should be pressing lightly into the ground (Fig. 37).
3. Move your legs downwards and towards the ground without your lower back coming away from it (Fig. 38); if it does, you can shorten the leg length by bringing them closer to your glutes (bottom) as you move them towards the ground.

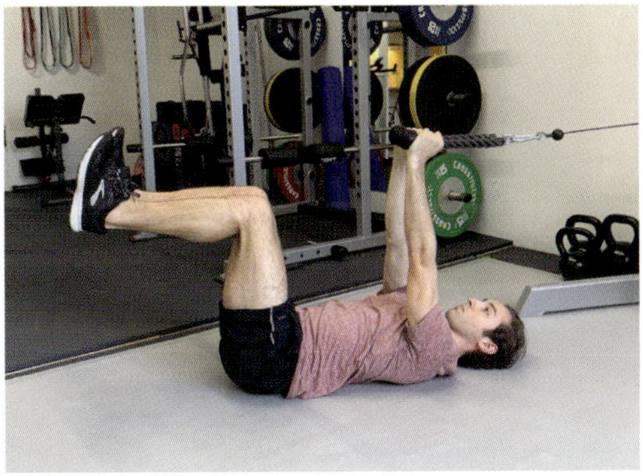

Fig. 37 Resisted dead bug start position.

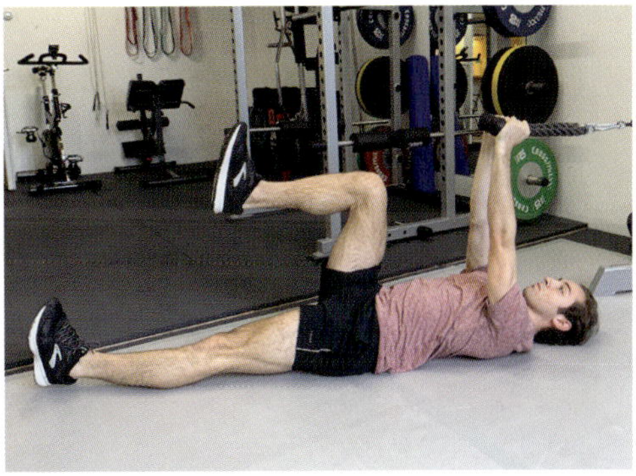

Fig. 38 Movement.

CORE EXERCISES

Forward ball rolls

This is an anti-extension exercise with the difference being that you are now using a slightly unstable object to move on.

1. Start on your knees and place your forearms on the apex of the ball, then raise your knees off the ground so that your legs are straight (Fig. 39).
2. Slowly roll the ball forward and out away from you. As you begin the movement, be sure to squeeze your glutes tightly as this will prevent you from going into extension. Only roll out as far as you can while maintaining good form otherwise you will feel this in your back and not your stomach (Fig. 40).
3. Once you have reached your outermost point roll the ball back towards yourself.

Stir the pot

A slightly more advanced version than a plank and forward ball roll, this exercise challenges the 'core' in a great way and can be scaled to be more difficult by increasing the circle you make while performing this.

1. Start up on your toes with your legs spread a little in order to maintain a good stable position.
2. Place the ball under your chest with your forearms placed on top of the ball. Push yourself up and away from the ball, bracing your core and squeezing your glutes (Fig. 41).
3. Start to make small circles clockwise for the required number of repetitions and then repeat counter-clockwise.

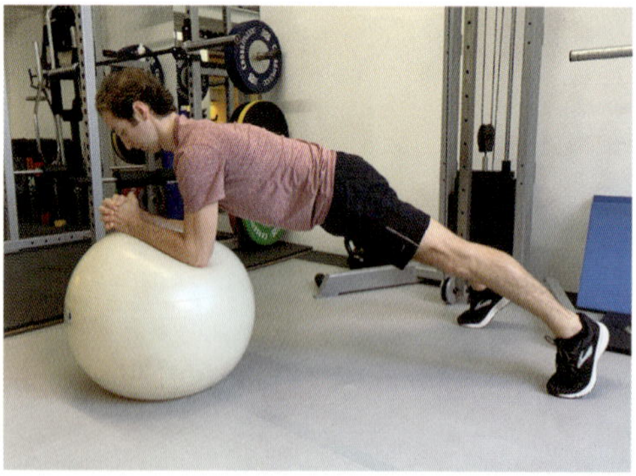

Fig. 39 Start position for forward ball rolls.

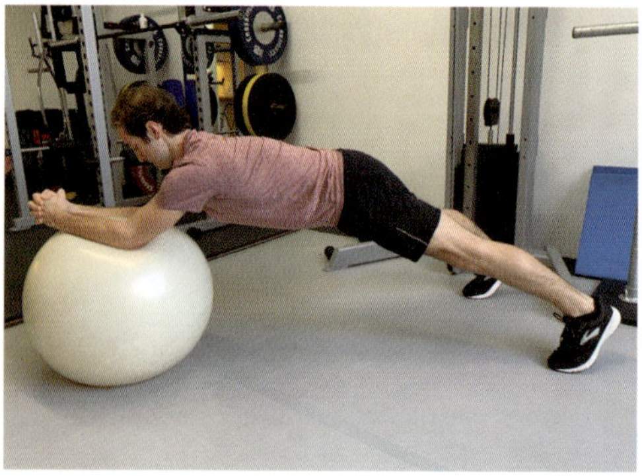

Fig. 40 Movement.

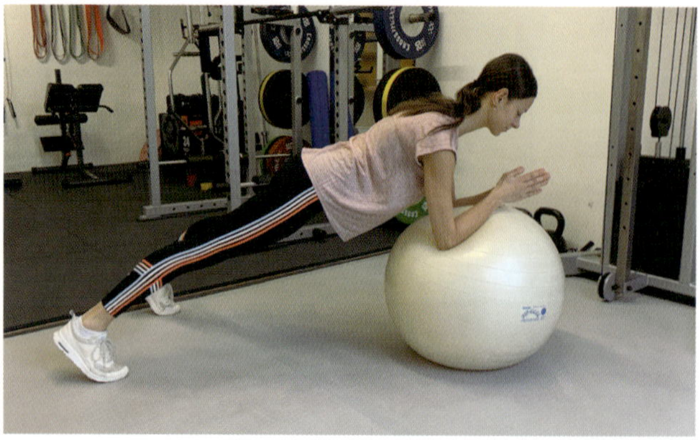

Fig. 41 Stir the pot position.

Plank

The plank is one of the most well-known but incorrectly used exercises. It is part of the anti-extension exercises and helps with learning to engage not only the anterior part of your core but also your glutes.

1. Starting in a quadruped position, place your elbows on the ground in line with your shoulders and move your legs straight out behind you, keeping your hips from sinking downwards.
2. Squeeze your glutes together and brace your abdominals. Make sure to push through your shoulder blades to activate your serratus anterior.
3. Your body should be in an almost straight line (Fig. 42).

Reverse planks

This is a much harder variation of the standard plank and therefore falls into the anti-extension bracket. As the hips are in an extended position and fighting against gravity it teaches you how to stay tight in an extended position (much as the standard plank, just much harder). This carries over well to dance where overhead lifts and jumps are involved.

Depending on the equipment available you need to be able to fixate your ankles and create space just above your hips; a glute ham developer is ideal for this.

1. Place your ankles between the foot pads and your hips just over the fulcrum of the large pad.
2. Lower yourself backwards until you are lying almost horizontally and hold in that position.
3. Keep a slight bend in the knees and do not go too far backwards otherwise you will feel it in your back (Fig. 43).
4. There are many ways to increase the difficulty of this exercise, such as using the arms to create a longer lever (Figs 44 and 45), or for an even harder version, a single leg.

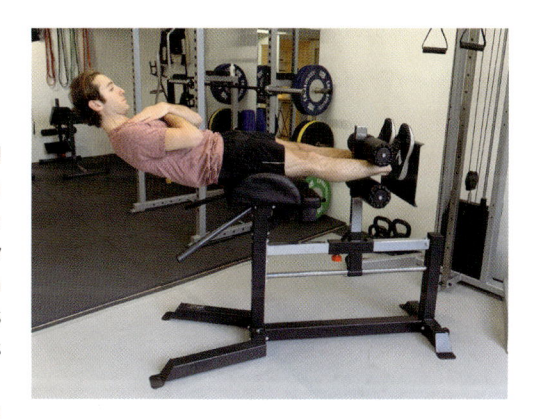

Fig. 43 Reverse plank position.

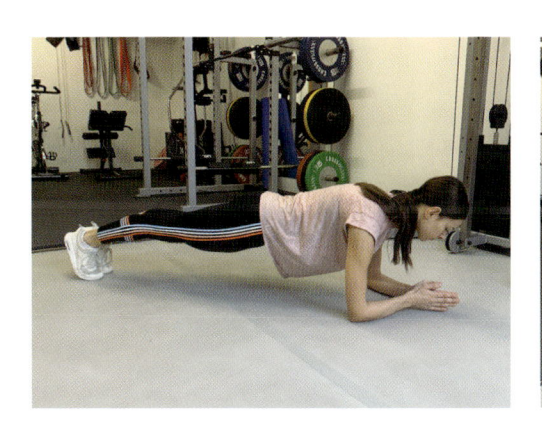

Fig. 42 Plank position.

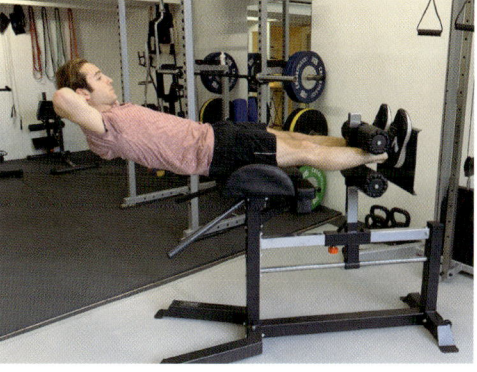

Fig. 44 Extended arms 1.

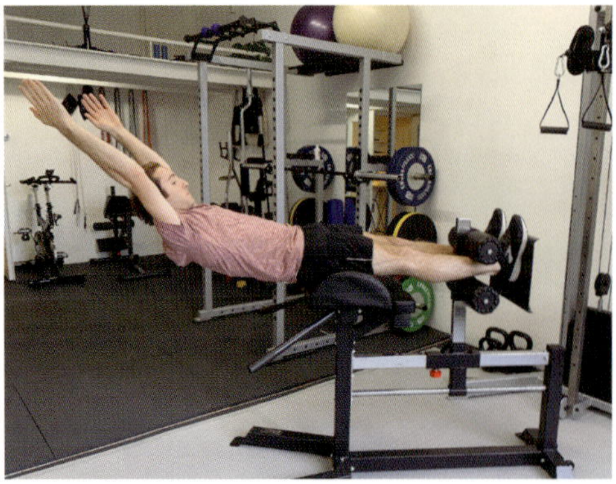

CORE EXERCISES

Fig. 45 Extended arms 2.

Side plank

The side plank is what is known as an anti-lateral flexion exercise. To hold this position you must use your obliques and quadratus lumborum to prevent yourself from collapsing sideways. This in turn will strengthen the aforementioned musculature, a very often neglected but highly important muscle group for creating a strong core, which in turn will create good spinal stability.

1. Lying on your side the first thing you must do is set the shoulder girdle in place so that the scapula is locked and can be used as a good solid base to push away from.
2. Your ankles, knees, hip, shoulders and ears should all line up (Fig. 46).
3. Once this is established, raise your hips from the ground while activating your glutes to stop yourself from sinking backwards until you are in a completely straight line, and hold (Fig. 47).
4. You can do this for time or repetitions.

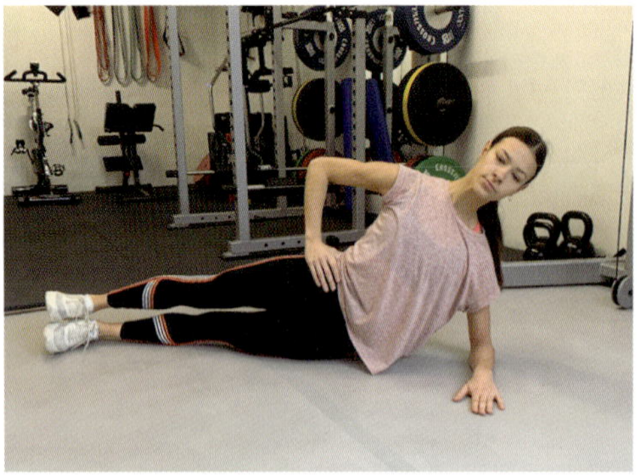

Fig. 46 Side plank start position.

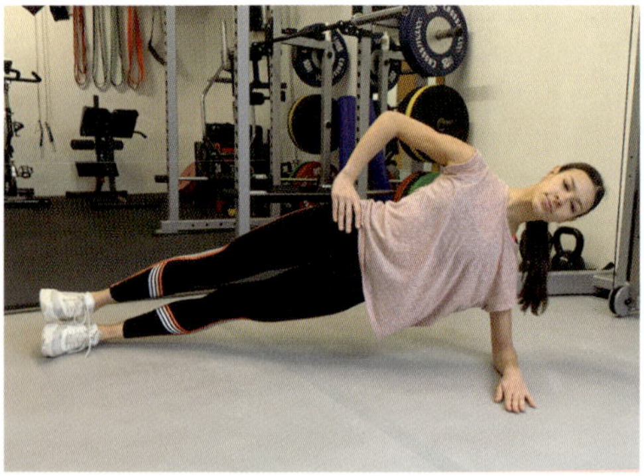

Fig. 47 Side plank hold position.

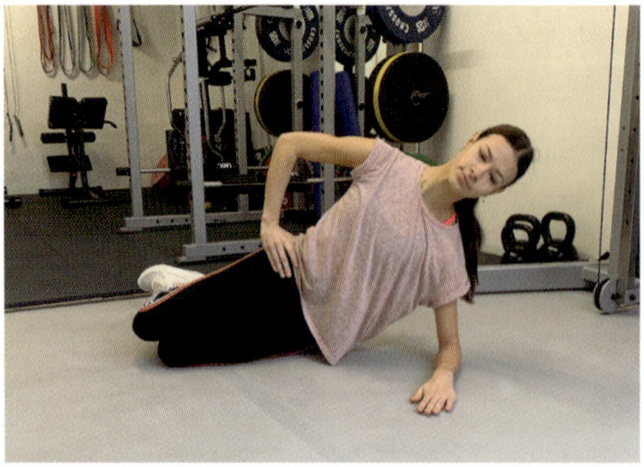

Fig. 48 Modified start position.

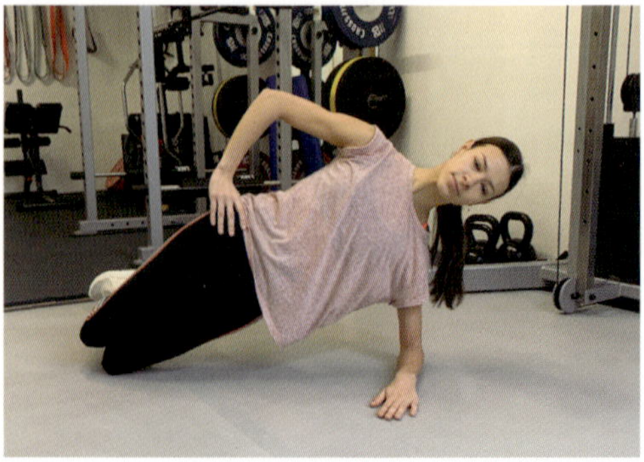

Fig. 49 Modified hold position.

CORE EXERCISES

5. An easier version is where you bend your legs to a 90-degree angle and do it from the knees (Figs 48 and 49).

Side plank with band for gluteus medius

Adding a band to this exercise allows you to recruit the gluteus medius muscle which is an external rotator of the hip and helps with knee alignment. It also has the added bonus of becoming a more unstable exercise allowing for greater recruitment of the trunk musculature.

1. The easiest version of this is to begin with the plank variation on the knees and then place a band just above the knees (to make it harder you can place it below the knees).

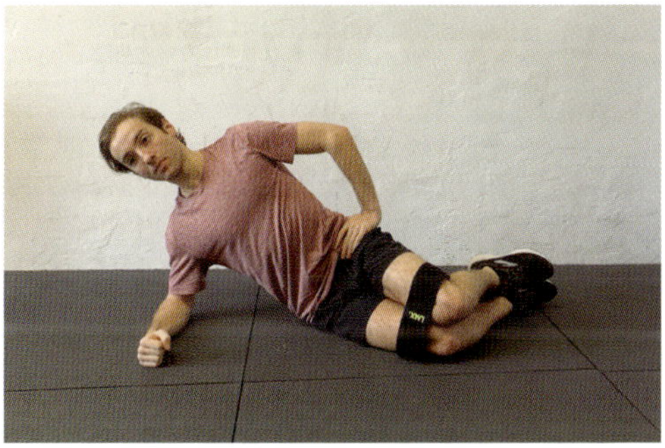

Fig. 50 Side plank with glute engagement.

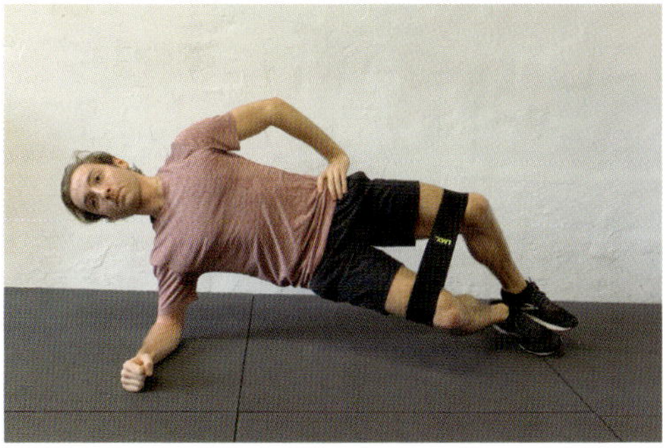

Fig. 51 Movement.

2. Set yourself up exactly like in a side plank on the knees (Fig. 50).
3. Once in position raise yourself up off the ground and open the outer leg against the band (Fig. 51).
4. This can be performed for time or repetitions.
5. A progression of this would be to perform it with the legs straight and opening up the top leg pushing it against the band.

Copenhagen side plank

This variation of the side plank helps to strengthen the adductors alongside the obliques and quadratus lumborum.

1. Begin by placing one leg bent at a 90-degree angle under a bench and the other on top (Fig. 52).
2. Get the rest of your body set up as in the other side plank variations.
3. Lift your hips up and lift the leg up that is on the ground and squeeze it into the underside of the bench (Fig. 53).
4. This can be performed for time or repetitions.
5. The more advanced version is with the legs straight (Fig. 54).

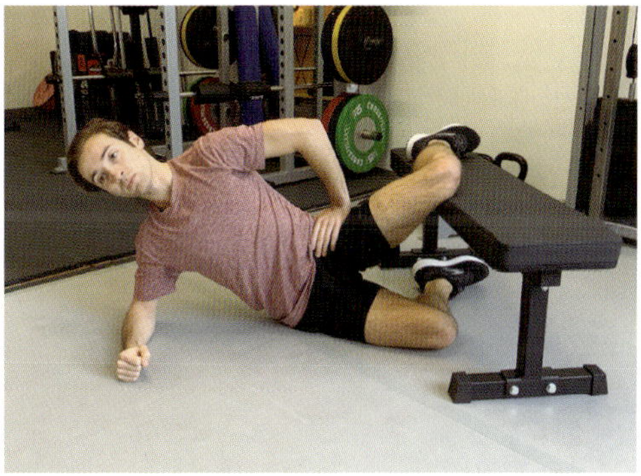

Fig. 52 Copenhagen side plank start position.

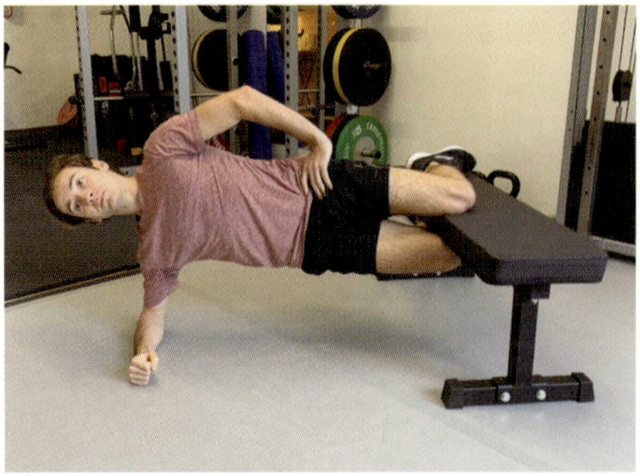

CORE EXERCISES

Fig. 53 Copenhagen side plank hold position.

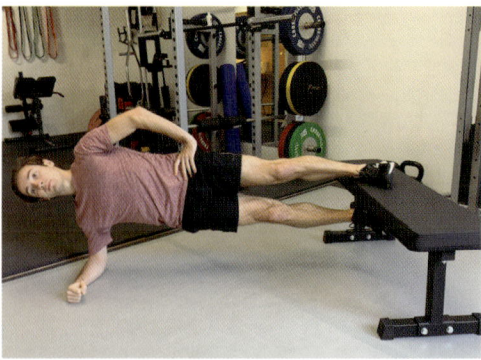

Fig. 54 Copenhagen side plank advanced position.

Bird-dog

This exercise is to teach hip back disassociation without using the ground as a contact point such as in the dead-bug. It can also be used to help people find their neutral pelvic alignment and aid in being able to maintain this through a movement.

1. Get down on the ground into a quadruped position (hands and knees). Your knees should be in line with your hip at a 90-degree angle and your wrists in line with your shoulder. Your elbows should be pointing backwards and you should be pushing yourself away through your mid-back so that you engage your serratus anterior (Fig. 55).
2. Move one leg and the opposite arm away from your midline, make sure that your thumb is pointing upwards as this will create more space in the shoulder by externally rotating it.
3. Your leg should finish parallel to the ground and your arm in line with your ear (Fig. 56).

Be sure that there is no movement in the trunk at all. This exercise can easily be regressed by taking away the movement of one of the extremities. It can also be progressed by raising the knees off the ground.

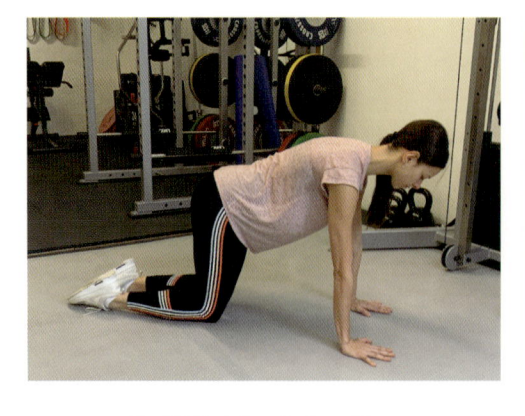

Fig. 55 Bird-dog start position.

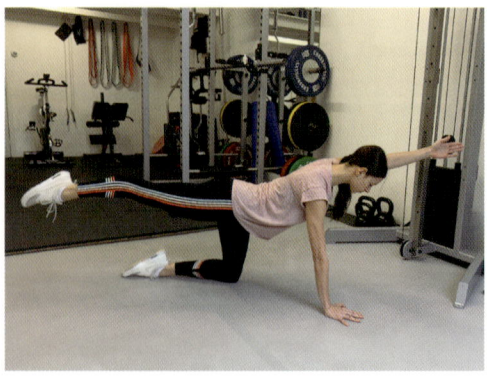

Fig. 56 Movement.

CORE EXERCISES

Bird dog with stability ball against wall

This variation is to increase intra-abdominal pressure.

1. Place a ball behind you against a wall.
2. Assume the same position as the standard bird-dog (Fig. 57), with the exception that you will raise your knees slightly off the ground and push back against the ball and hold for a count of up to 10 seconds (Fig. 58).

To increase the difficulty, you can simply take one arm off the ground, while holding and then repeat with the other arm (Fig. 59).

Bear crawls

The bear crawl is the locomotive version of the bird-dog which helps continue to teach corset control while moving.

1. Start in a quadruped position and raise your knees off the ground (Fig. 60).
2. Move your hands and feet in opposition to go forwards all the while maintaining trunk stability (Figs 61 and 62).

A good external feedback aid is to place a water bottle that is laid down on your lower back and then move forwards without letting the bottle fall. Do this exercise for time rather than repetitions.

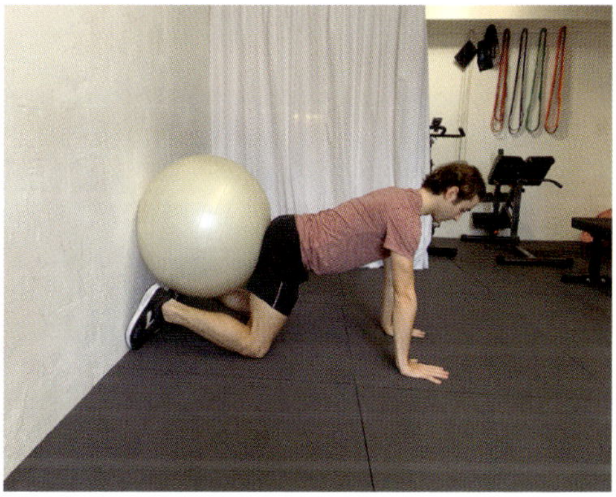

Fig. 57 Bird-dog with stability ball start position.

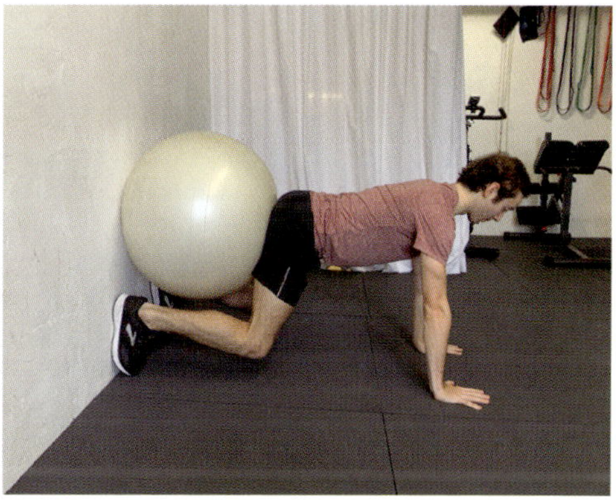

Fig. 58 Movement.

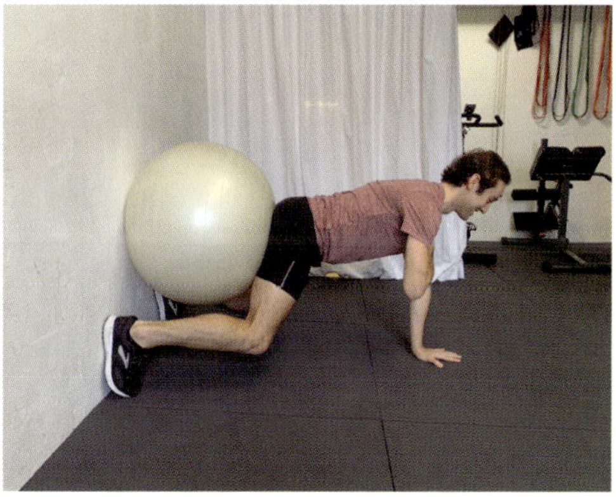

Fig. 59 Advanced bird-dog version.

83

CORE EXERCISES

Fig. 60 Bear crawl start position.

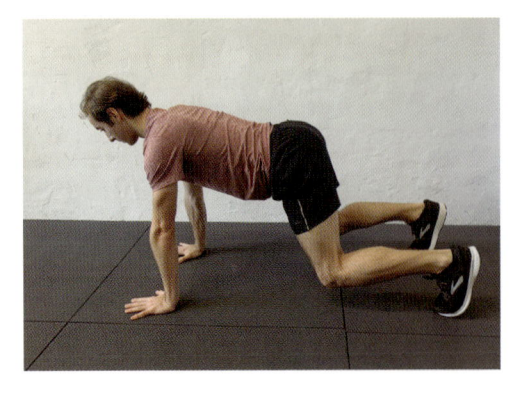

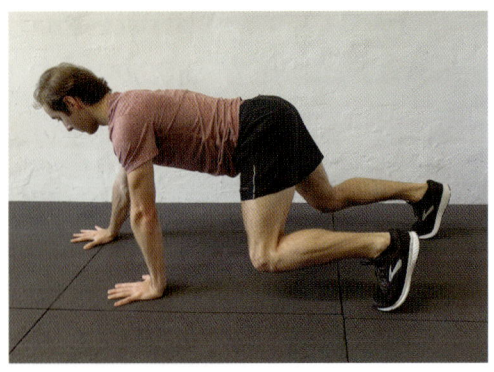

Fig. 61 Movement.

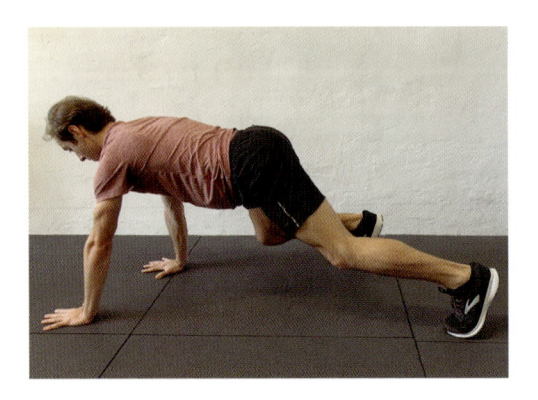

Fig. 62 Movement progression.

Suitcase carries

This is a very simple and great dynamic exercise that strengthens the obliques and quadratus lumborum and you can use a variety of implements from kettlebells to barbells to sandbags for this exercise.

1. Start by selecting the object that you want to lift at the appropriate weight to be lifted.
2. Lower yourself into position to pick the weight up in one hand and lift (Fig. 63).
3. You will then carry the weight (Fig. 64), for a given amount of time or distance before switching sides and repeating.

Half kneeling Pallof press

The half kneeling Pallof press is an anti-rotation exercise, meaning that you have to resist against an external force trying to rotate the spine with whichever device is used throughout. It is a great way to start to integrate the brace in an upright position and maintain trunk stiffness. This helps with being able to transfer power from the lower extremities through to the upper ones, such as when partnering.

1. Position the cable at the height of your solar plexus when on your knee.
2. Make sure to be on the knee closest to the cable with the knee on the ground in line with your hip. Your other leg should be at

CORE EXERCISES

Fig. 63 Suitcase carry start position.

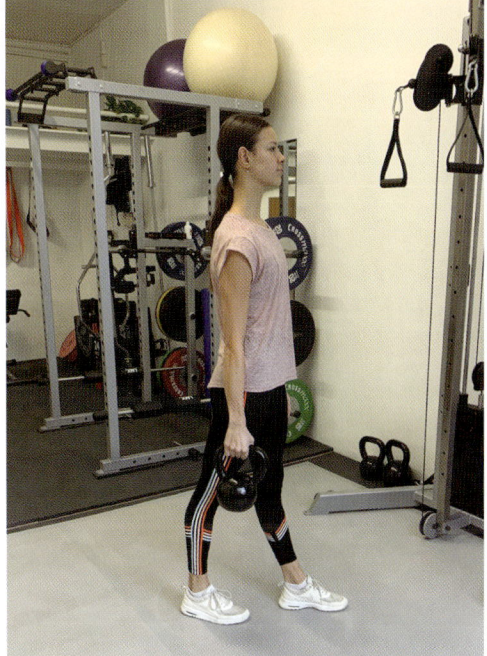

Fig. 64 Movement.

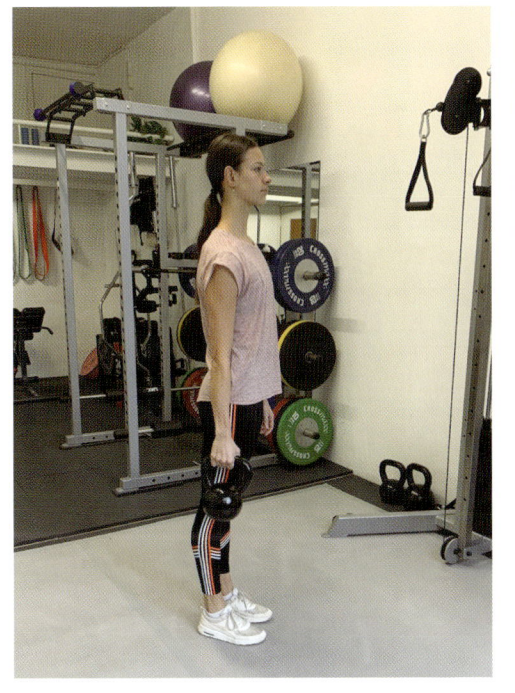

a 90-degree angle at the hip and knee with the whole foot on the ground.
3. Take the handle in your hands with one hand over the other and pull the cable towards your centre with your arms bent (Fig. 65).
4. Take a breath, brace your stomach, activate your glutes, then straighten your arm out in front of you (Fig. 66), while letting your breath out through pursed lips.
5. Bring your arms back in again and repeat.

There are many, many ways to perform this exercise and this is just one of them.

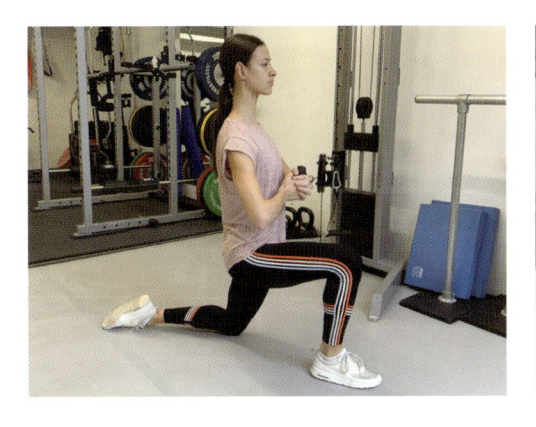

Fig. 65 Half kneeling Pallof press start position.

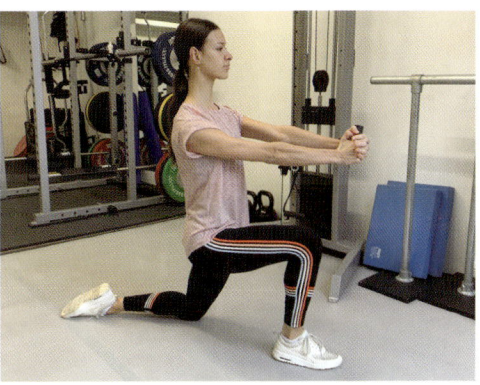

Fig. 66 Movement.

85

CORE EXERCISES

Standing Pallof press

1. Position the cable at the height of the solar plexus.
2. Stand in profile to the cable machine with your feet in a wide stance. This ensures that the hips are locked in place and you have a good sturdy base to commence the exercise with.
3. Place your hands with one over the other around the cable attachment and pull it towards your midline (Fig. 67).
4. Take a breath, brace your stomach, squeeze your glutes and straighten your arms in front of you (Fig. 68), at the same time letting your breath out through pursed lips (this is known as a partial Valsalva manoeuvre).
5. Bring your arms back in and repeat.

There are many small changes that you can make to this exercise to make it harder or easier.

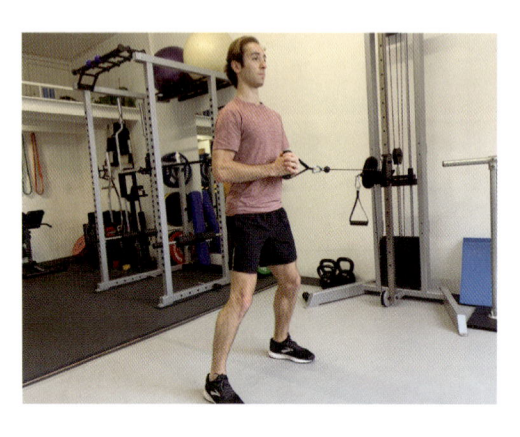

Fig. 67 Standing Pallof start position.

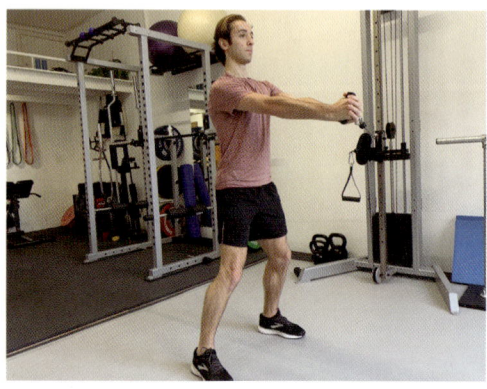

Fig. 68 Movement.

7 | LOWER-BODY EXERCISES

The majority of exercises included here are closed kinetic chain movements across multiple joints, using multiple muscles. They range between single-leg and combined leg exercises to provide variety as well as challenging possible bilateral deficiencies.

UNILATERAL KNEE DOMINANT

Step-ups (differing heights)

For step-ups and their variations, the primary focus is on the quadriceps and gluteus maximus; the gluteus medius plays a role in keeping the hips and knees in line throughout the movement. These exercises are good to help people who have a hard time keeping their knees from falling inwards.

In this version we are performing a lateral step-up.

1. Place your foot on the step in a comfortable position. The step should be just below knee height at mid-shin level. The other foot should be in a fully flexed position with the toes pointing upwards; this takes away the possibility to push off from the toes throughout the exercise (Fig. 69).
2. Begin by driving up with the working leg, push through the whole foot (heel and forefoot), as this will help to engage the glutes (Fig. 70).
3. Keep the hips square throughout the movement.
4. Lower in the same manner and repeat for the required number of repetitions.

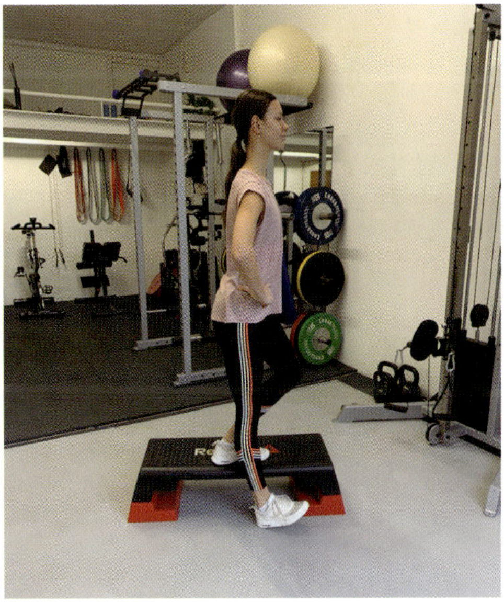

Fig. 69 Step-up start position.

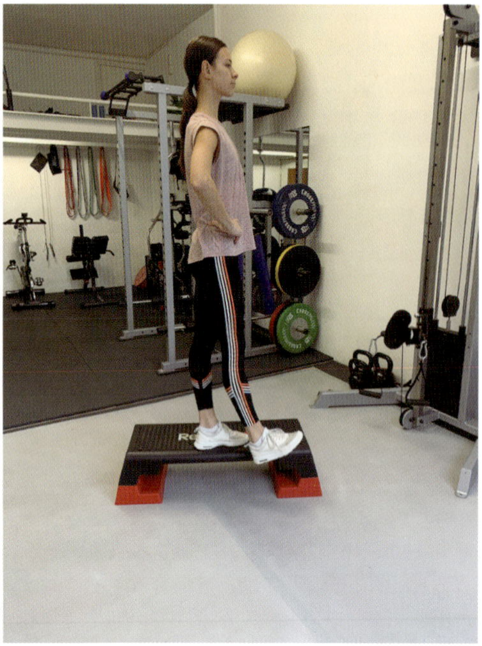

LOWER-BODY EXERCISES

Skater squat

The skater squat is in essence a step-up; don't be fooled by its simplicity, however, as it is a very difficult exercise to perform correctly. The reason for this is that it takes away any impetus used by the non-working side to help with the working leg.

1. Start in a half kneeling position and place a pad under the knee of the non-working leg to avoid banging down on it (once you have the hang of the exercise you can take it away) (Fig. 71).
2. Place your arms in front of you and then lean your bodyweight forward over the working leg and, without using the back leg, lift yourself up (Fig. 72).
3. Once in the top position begin to lower yourself down to your starting position.
4. Repeat for the required number of repetitions.

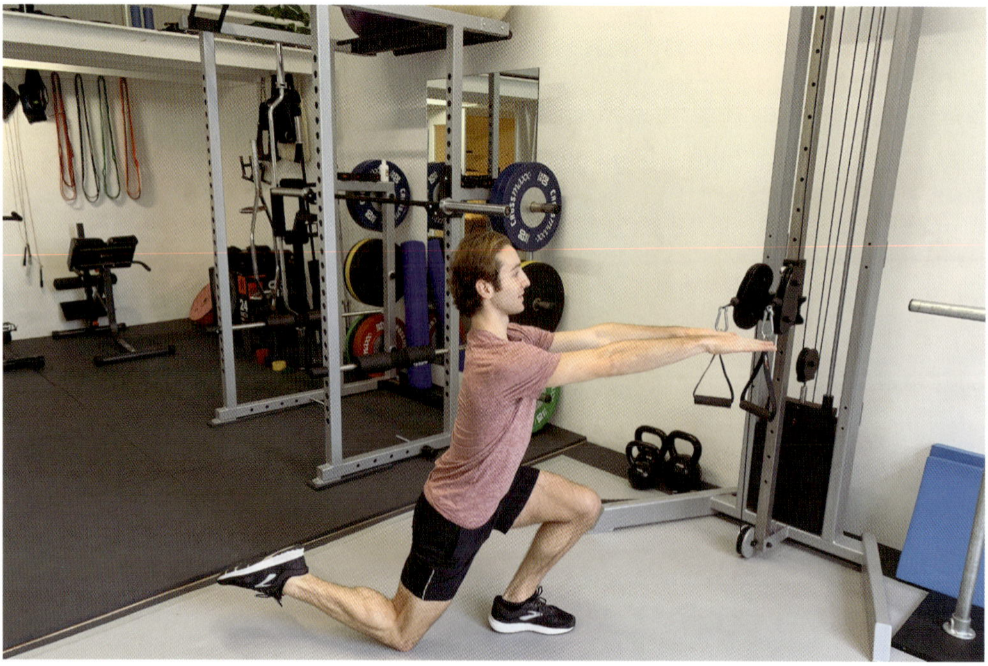

Fig. 70 Movement.

Fig. 71 Skater squat start position.

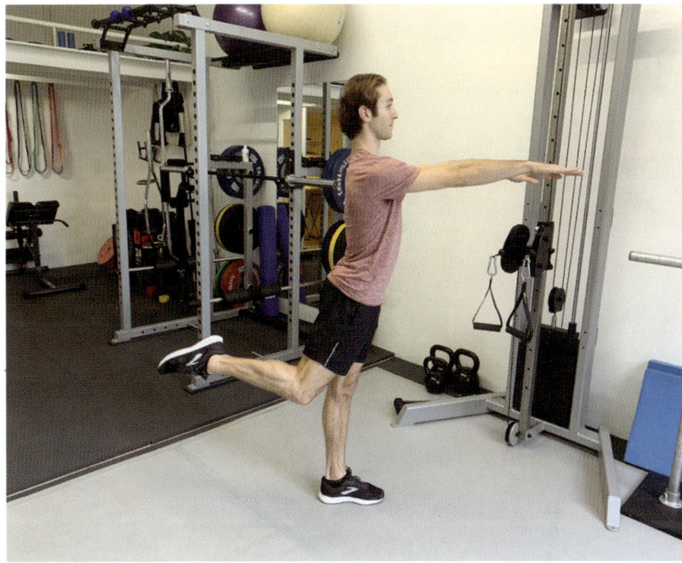

LOWER-BODY EXERCISES

Fig. 72 Movement.

To increase the difficulty, you can place your hands across your chest and then behind your head, you can then increase the range of motion by adding a small step under the working foot.

Shrimps

The shrimp is just a more advanced version of a skater squat – the difference being that you now hold the non-working leg with your hands (Fig. 73).

1. Start with one hand holding the leg and one arm in front, lean your body forward over the working leg and lift yourself up (Fig. 74).
2. You can slowly progress this to holding the leg with both hands by firstly bringing the arm in front of you to across the chest, then behind your head, and finally holding the leg.

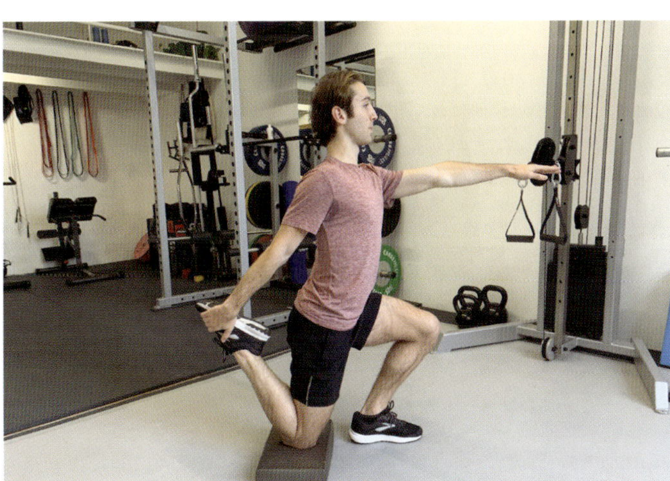

Fig. 73 Shrimp starting position.

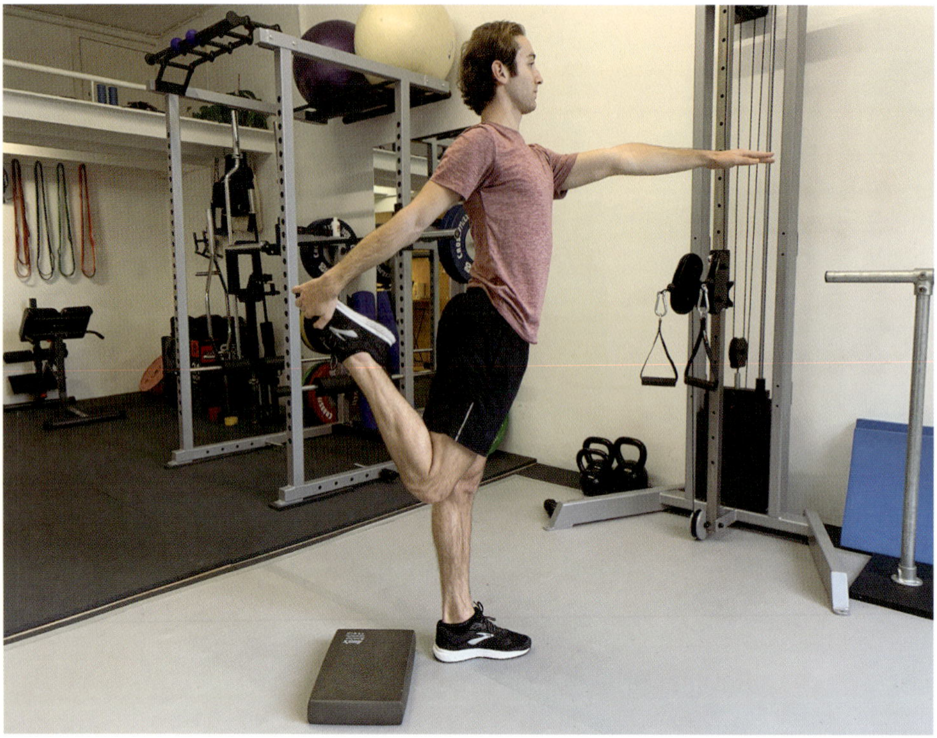

LOWER-BODY EXERCISES

Fig. 74 Movement.

SPLIT SQUAT VARIATIONS

The split squat and its variations are extremely versatile exercises, as you can make them easier or harder by changing implements (dumbbells, barbells, kettlebells, bands), positions of the implements (in front, on the back, by the side), the plane of motion (sagittal, frontal), and by raising the working or non-working leg to increase range of motion. They are a fantastic way to introduce lower body training, coming with a big 'bang for your buck' and helping to even out imbalances between the right and left sides.

Front foot elevated split squats

1. Place a foot on the step in a split stance; your back leg should be far enough away from you so that your heel is off the ground and your feet should be hip-width apart so that you create a good base to begin from (Fig. 75).
2. When you begin your descent, think about going down in a diagonal and not in a straight line. Your knee (if it is healthy), should travel past your toes to a point just before the heel of the working leg starts to rise. Your back leg should remain slightly bent throughout the movement (Fig. 76).
3. When you begin to come back to your starting point from the bottom position, make sure to push through the heel of your working leg so that you can use your glutes.

Split squats

1. Get into a split stance just far enough apart so that the heel of your back leg comes

LOWER-BODY EXERCISES

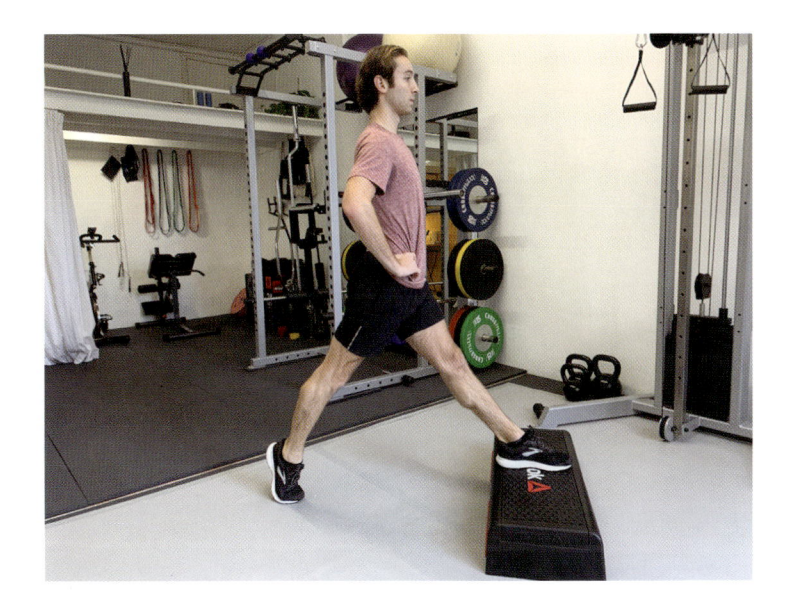

Fig. 75 Front foot elevated split squat start position.

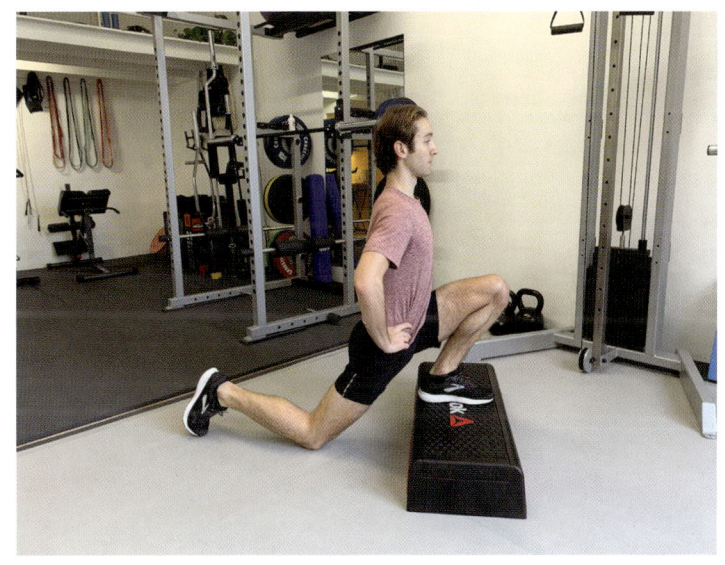

Fig. 76 Movement.

up. Your feet should be hip-width apart to create a good stable base (Fig. 77).

2. When you begin your descent, think about going down in a diagonal and not in a straight line. Your knee (if it is healthy), should travel past your toes to a point just before the heel of the working leg starts to rise. Your back leg should remain slightly bent throughout the movement (Fig. 78).

3. When you begin to come back to your starting point from the bottom position, make sure to push through the heel of your working leg so that you can use your glutes.

4. Make sure that the knee of the working leg doesn't cave inwards or move too far outwards; it should track over the second toe.

LOWER-BODY EXERCISES

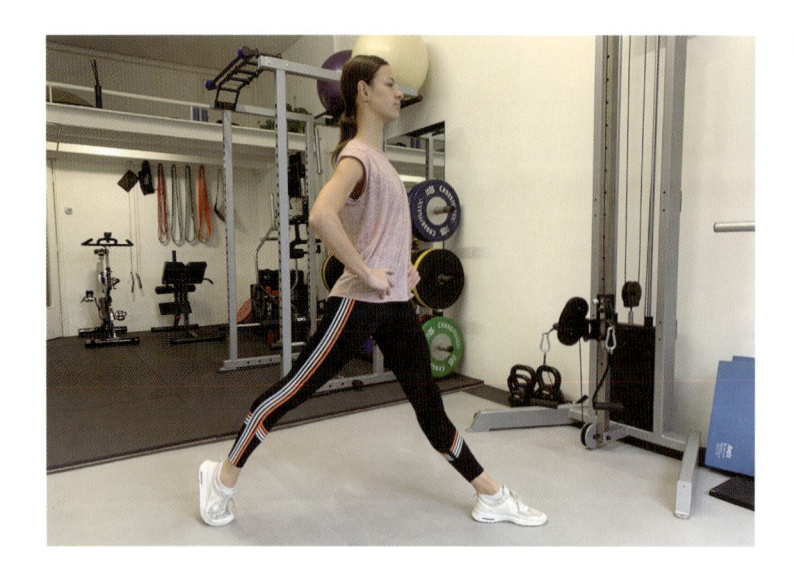

Fig. 77 Split squat start.

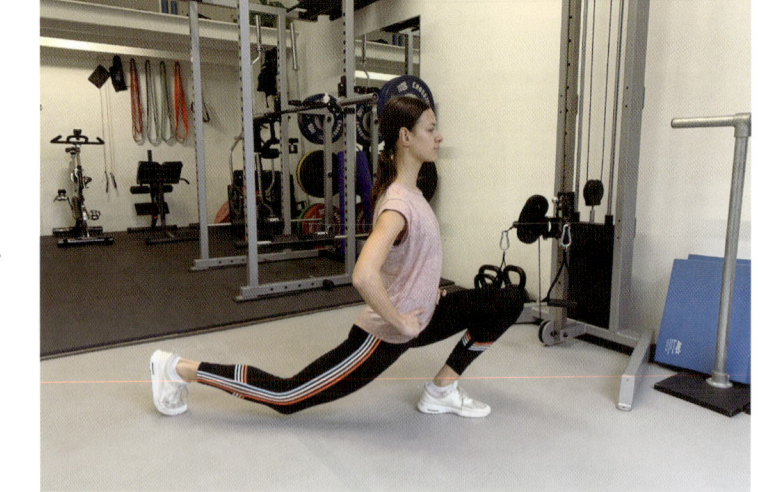

Fig. 78 Movement.

Lateral split squats

The lateral split squat focuses on strengthening the quadriceps, gluteus maximus and adductors and works within the frontal plane which is an often-neglected area when strength training for dance. You can use a wide variety of implements for this exercise, such as kettlebells, dumbbells, barbells, sandbags and waterbags to increase difficulty in numerous ways.

1. Begin in a wide stance with your feet outside of your shoulders and the toes pointing slightly outwards (Fig. 79).
2. Bend at the knee of the leg you want to work and slowly lower yourself until you have reached your end position then bring yourself back to where you began (Fig. 80).
3. You can either repeat on the same leg or do it with the opposing one. Repeat for the required number of repetitions.

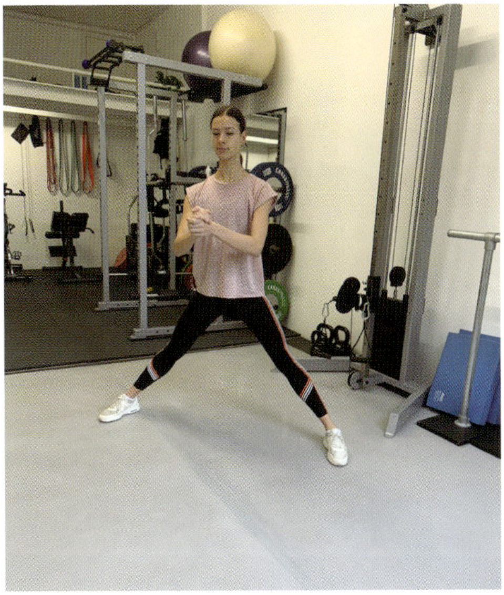

LOWER-BODY EXERCISES

Fig. 79 Lateral split squat start position.

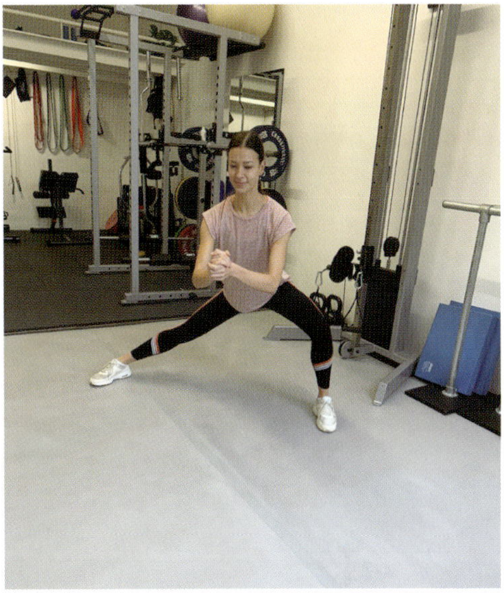

Fig. 80 Movement.

Rear foot elevated split squats
1. Stand facing away from a bench or step and place one foot on it. You may have to move the working leg forwards or backwards in order to find the right position; everyone is different, so this varies from person to person (Fig. 81).

2. When you begin your descent, think about going down in a diagonal, making sure not to rock backwards and sit in the bottom position, you must remain active during the entirety of the exercise (Fig. 82). Your knee (if it is healthy) will travel past your toes to a point just before the heel of the working

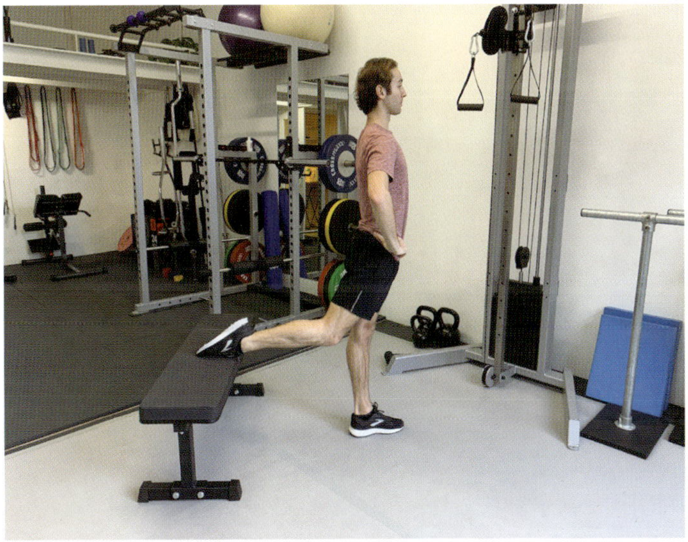

Fig. 81 Rear foot elevated split squat start position.

93

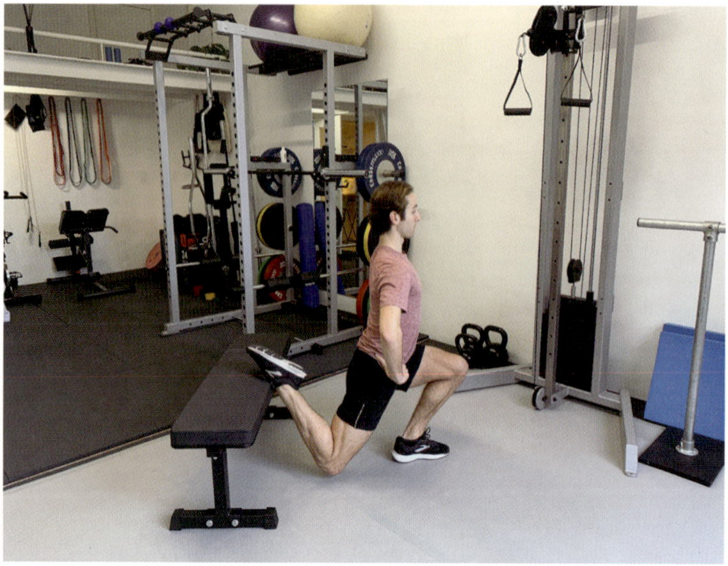

LOWER-BODY EXERCISES

Fig. 82 Movement.

leg starts to rise. Your back leg should remain bent throughout the movement.
3. When you begin to come back to your starting point from the bottom position, make sure to push through the heel of your working leg so that you can use your glutes.
4. Make sure that the working leg's knee doesn't cave inwards or move too far outwards, it should track over the second toe.

Lunges onto a step

This is the dynamic version of a split squat. By lunging onto a step, it decreases the impact on landing. This exercise strengthens the quadriceps, gluteus maximus and the adductors as they play a stabilizing role.

1. Before you begin, make sure to find the right distance by doing a split squat on the step first. Once you've done this you can begin (Fig. 83).
2. Lunge forward onto the step until you reach full depth. Your knee will travel past your toes (unless you've been told not to by a qualified healthcare practitioner).
3. When you push back, drive through the heel to activate the glutes and push yourself into the starting position.
4. Repeat on the opposing leg.

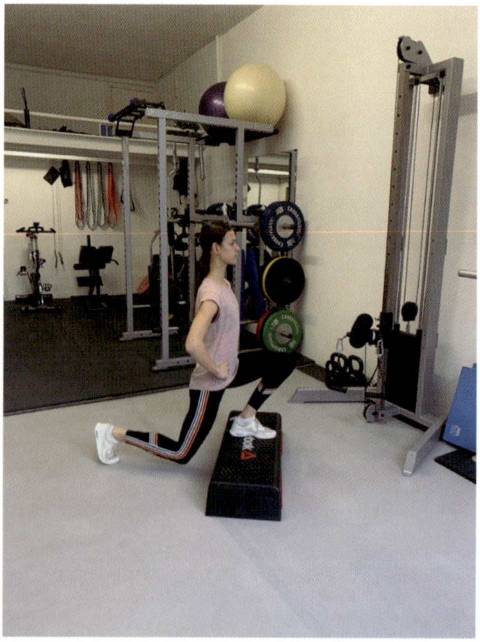

Fig. 83 Lunge onto step movement.

LOWER-BODY EXERCISES

5. Keep your core braced slightly throughout the exercise so that you don't break in the middle.
6. Repeat for the required number of repetitions.

Reverse lunges off a step

The backwards lunge off a step puts the emphasis on the leg that is on the step and not the one that is moving. It helps to strengthen the quadriceps and gluteus maximus.

1. Begin by using a low step and stand on it (Fig. 84).
2. Step backwards off the step until you have reached the correct depth for you (Fig. 85).
3. Then driving through the whole foot that is on the step bring yourself back to your starting position.
4. You can repeat on the same side or do this in an alternating fashion.

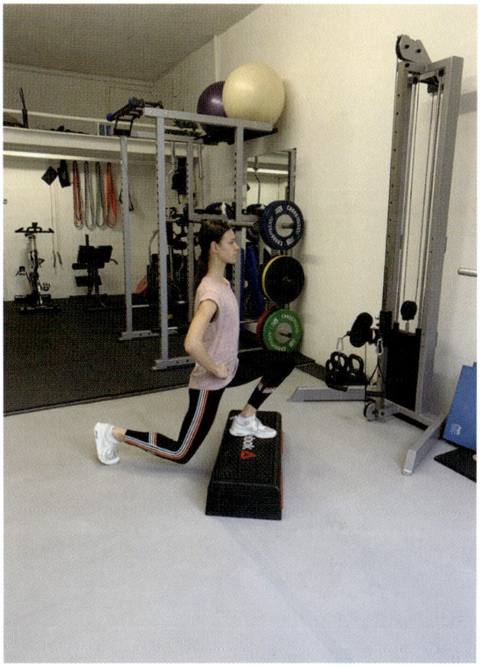

Fig. 85 Movement.

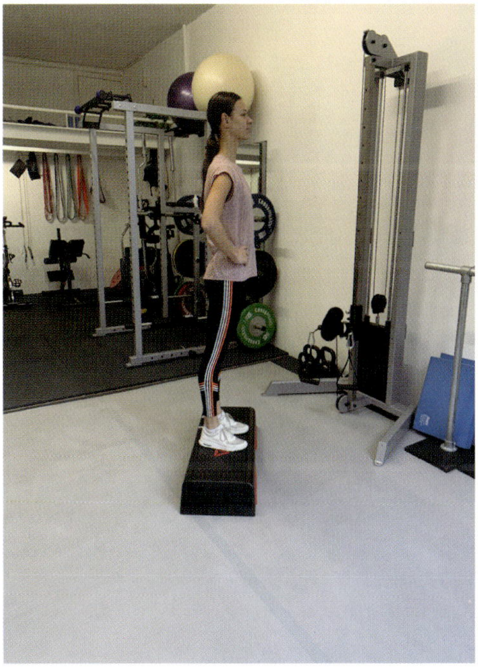

Fig. 84 Reverse lunges off a step start position.

Lateral lunges onto a step

This a great exercise and can be done as an active warm-up for those who may be a little tight in the adductors. As an exercise it helps to strengthen the quadriceps, adductors and gluteus maximus. There are many ways and many benefits of doing this exercise.

1. Before you begin, make sure to find the right distance by doing some lateral squats (Fig. 86).
2. Once you have found this, step out to the side; your toes will be pointing outwards and your body will naturally lean forward.
3. Make sure to land through the mid-foot and go through it until your heel touches the step (Fig. 87).
4. When returning to the beginning push through the toes and away from the working leg until you have returned to your starting point.

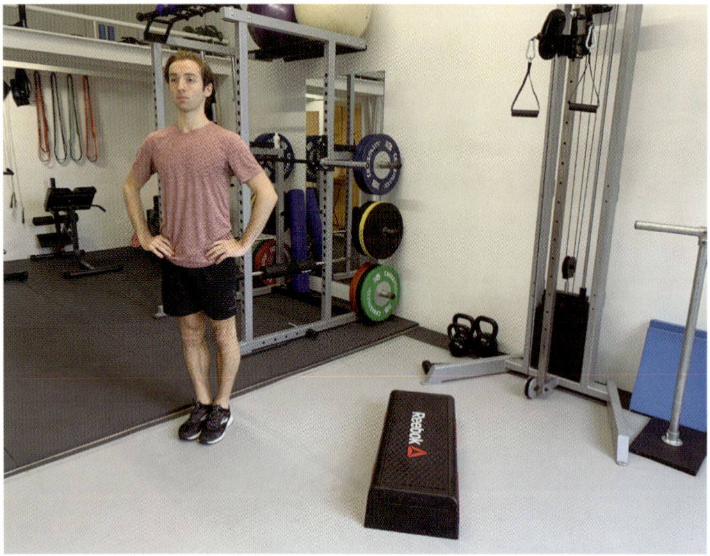

LOWER-BODY EXERCISES

Fig. 86 Lateral lunges onto a step start position.

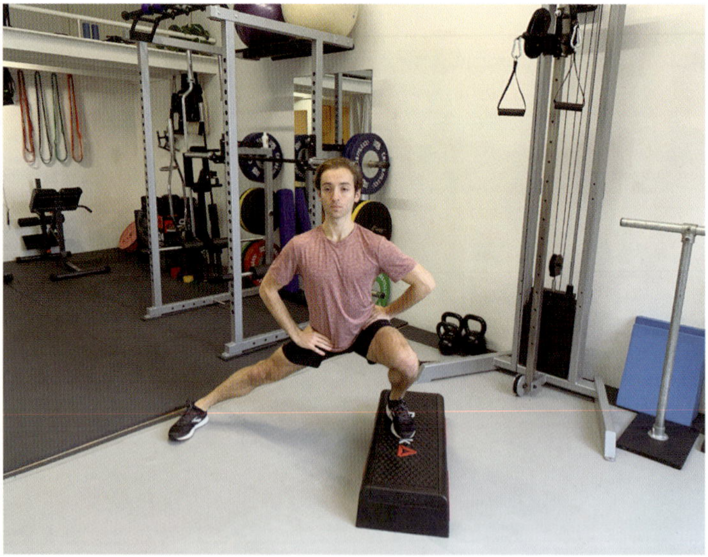

Fig. 87 Movement.

5. Keep your core braced slightly throughout the exercise.
6. Repeat for the required number of repetitions.

Walking lunges

Walking lunges can be done in numerous ways in order to place emphasis on certain muscles of the lower extremities. For example, making a short step places much more demand on the quadriceps, whereas making them long and wide places a greater demand on the adductors. You can use different implements and place them differently to increase or decrease demands.

1. Begin with your feet hip-width apart and holding the implement of choice (Fig. 88).

LOWER-BODY EXERCISES

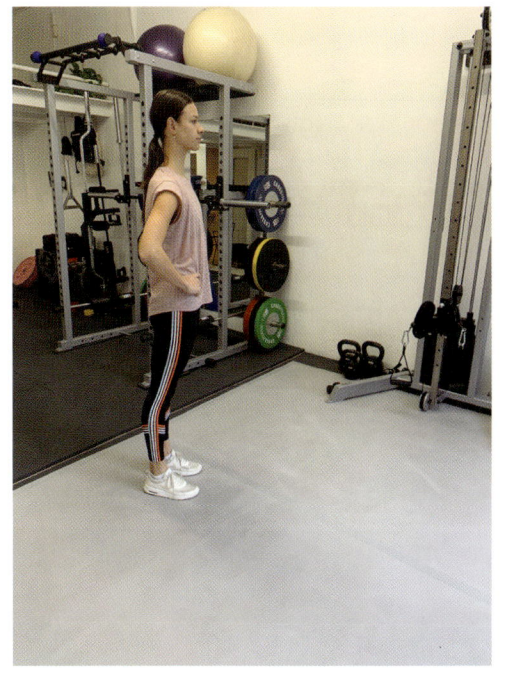

Fig. 88 Walking lunges start position.

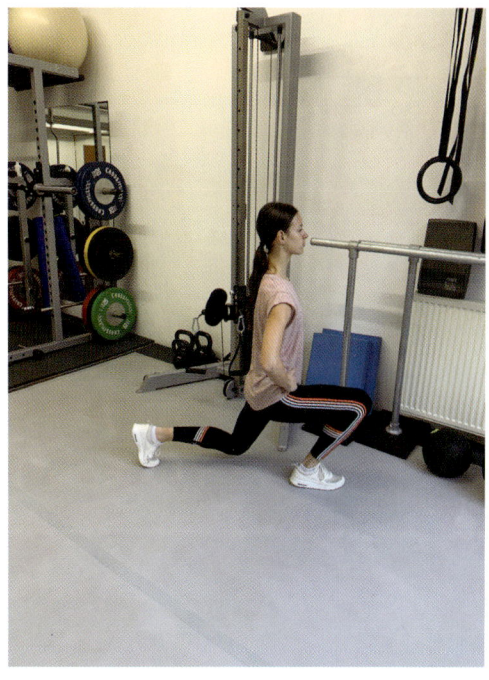

Fig. 90 End movement.

2. Take a step forward at the chosen width and stride length indicated and lower into your end range position (Fig. 89).
3. Push through the whole foot that has gone forward and drive yourself up and follow through with the next foot to take the next step (Fig. 90).
4. Repeat for the required number of repetitions.

Bilateral Knee Dominant

Bodyweight squat

This exercise is a great all-round exercise as it can be used as a warm-up, part of a mobility drill, and as a preparation tool before going into a workout. It works mainly the quadriceps, glutes and core.

1. Stand with your feet hip- or shoulder-width apart (this should feel comfortable for you), and your feet slightly turned out (Fig. 91).

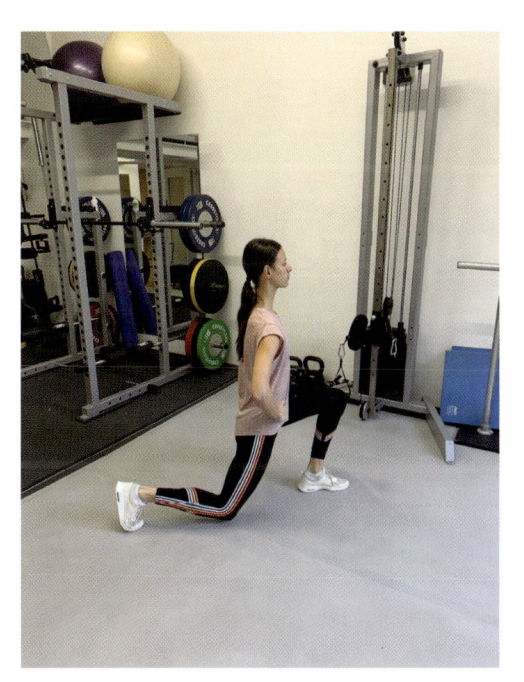

Fig. 89 Mid-movement.

97

LOWER-BODY EXERCISES

Fig. 91 Bodyweight squat start position.

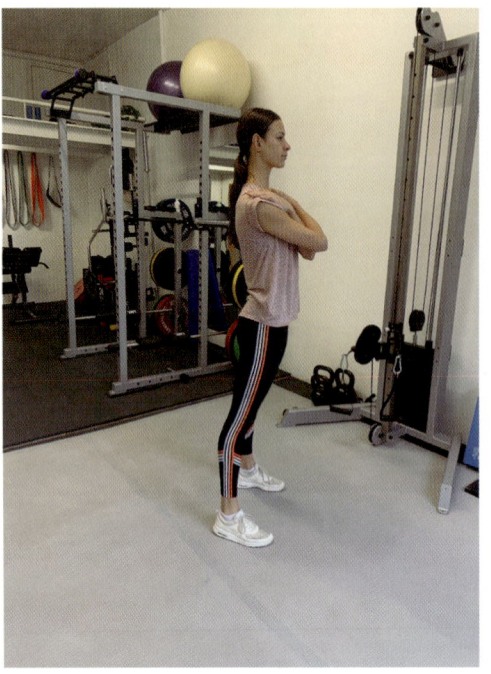

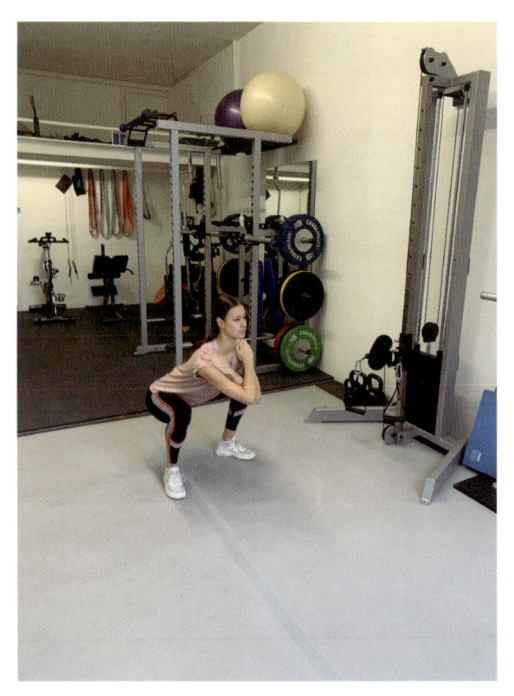

Fig. 92 Mid-movement.

2. Gently break at the knees and push your hips back as you descend.
3. Once you have reached the depth that is correct for you (Fig. 92), drive back up through the whole foot while squeezing your glutes.
4. You should be able to breathe through this exercise; however, make sure to keep a small amount of tension in your stomach (brace) throughout it.

Goblet squat

The goblet squat is a good exercise to help people keep upright during an exercise as the weight used pulls the person forward. It is also a precursor to the front squat and as an added bonus it is also a great assessment tool to see if someone is not utilizing their core correctly. (This can be seen when someone has what is known as a 'buttwink' during a bodyweight squat; if you give this exercise directly afterwards and the 'buttwink' is reduced and in some cases completely gone, it means that they are not holding enough tension in their core musculature.)

1. Choose your dumbbell or kettlebell and hold it against your chest (Fig. 93).
2. Stand with your feet hip- or shoulder-width apart (this should feel comfortable for you), and your feet slightly turned out.
3. Take a breath and brace your core, then, gently break at the knees and push your hips back as you descend.
4. Once you have reached the depth that is correct for you (Fig. 94), drive back up through the whole foot and squeeze your glutes, while letting your breath out through pursed lips, this is known as a partial Valsalva manoeuvre and helps to maintain your brace throughout the exercise.
5. Once you have reached the top take another breath and repeat the whole process.

LOWER-BODY EXERCISES

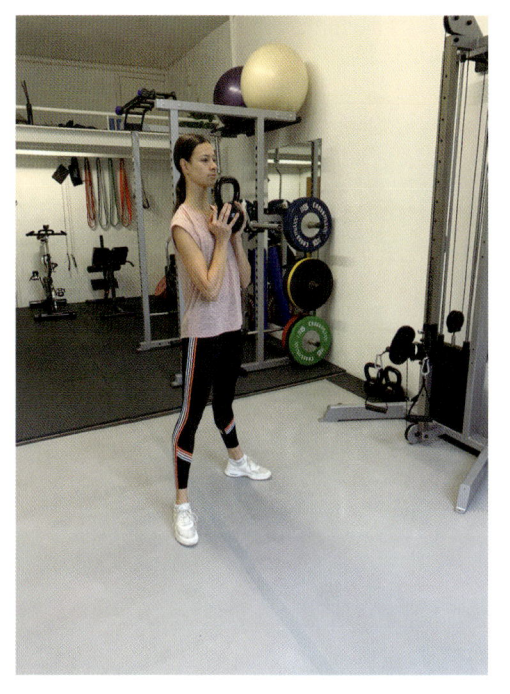

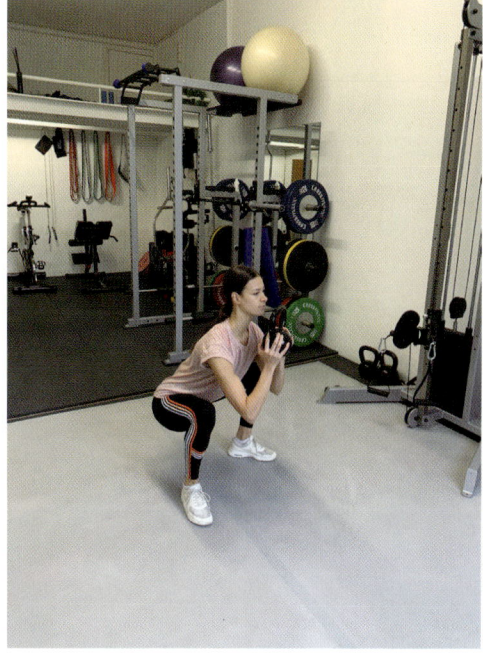

Fig. 93 Goblet squat start position.

Fig. 94 Mid-movement.

Trap-bar squat

The trap bar is an extremely versatile piece of equipment to have as it can be used for both squats and deadlifts by making the movement either more knee dominant or more hip dominant. For the squat variation this is a great way to introduce heavier load due to the position of the handles being by the side; this enables the person to be more upright and the spine in a more stacked position, therefore more spine sparing (friendly).

1. Stand inside the trap bar with your feet hip- or shoulder-width apart (this should feel comfortable for you), and your feet slightly turned out.
2. Break at the knees and push your hips back to go down. Take the handles on either side, lock your lats by pulling up against the handles but not actually lifting the weight, imagine also that you are pulling the bar behind you a little; you should now be in your squat position (Fig. 95).

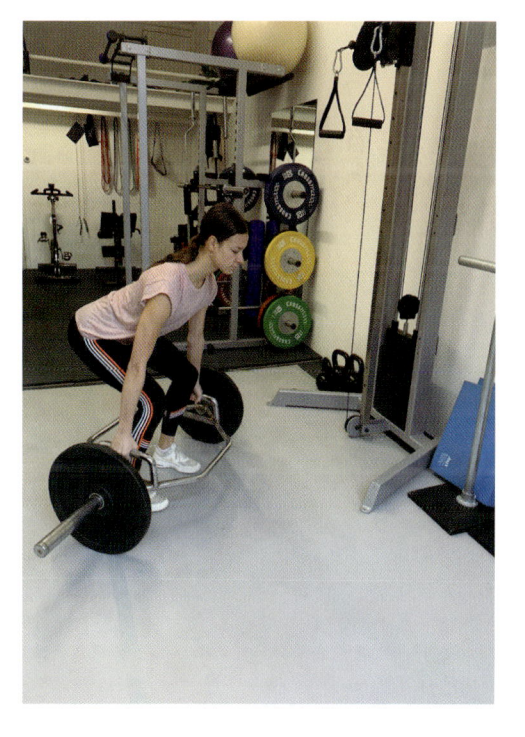

Fig. 95 Trap-bar squat start position.

LOWER-BODY EXERCISES

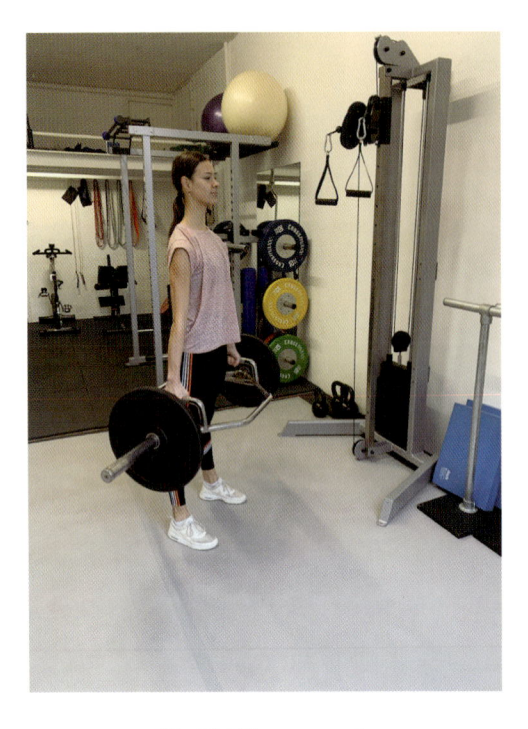

Fig. 96 Mid-movement.

3. Take a breath and brace your core, then drive up through the whole foot and squeeze your glutes.
4. Once at the top you can either take another breath or continue to hold as you lower the bar back down to the ground (Fig. 96).
5. Repeat the process for the required number of repetitions.

Front squat

The front squat is a good indicator of thoracic mobility and mid-back strength due to how the bar is positioned in front, because if there isn't enough of either the bar will slide forward.

It is a more spine sparing lift than the back squat as it allows you to be in a more upright position (stacked). It primarily works the quadriceps and glutes; however, it works a lot of other secondary muscles making it a good full body exercise.

1. The bar should be set in the pins at just below shoulder level (Fig. 97). This allows the person performing the squat to clear the pins when un-racking and re-racking the bar.
2. Once this has been done, stand in front of the bar, walk towards it and place the bar on top of your clavicular joint on the throat; this does not feel comfortable to start, but with time it gets easier.
3. Place your hands on the bar just outside of shoulder width and turn your elbows up towards the ceiling so that they are pointing out in front of you (Fig. 98).
4. If the arm position is too uncomfortable you can have your arms straight in front of you (also known as a zombie squat, Fig. 99), or take a crossed arm stance instead (Fig. 100).
5. Your feet should be hip- or shoulder-width apart (this should feel comfortable for you), and your feet slightly turned out.
6. Take a breath.
7. Lift the bar out of the rack and take one step back (Fig. 101).
8. Exhale through pursed lips then take another breath.
9. Break at the knees and push your hips back as you descend (Fig. 102).
10. Once you have reached the depth that is correct for you, drive back up through the whole foot and squeeze your glutes, while letting your breath out through pursed lips (this is known as a partial Valsalva manoeuvre and helps to maintain your brace throughout the exercise).
11. Once you have reached the top, take another breath and repeat the whole process.
12. When you have completed the required number of repetitions, re-rack the bar by taking a step towards the squat rack and imagine walking through it so that the bar touches the pins, making it safe for you to place it properly.

LOWER-BODY EXERCISES

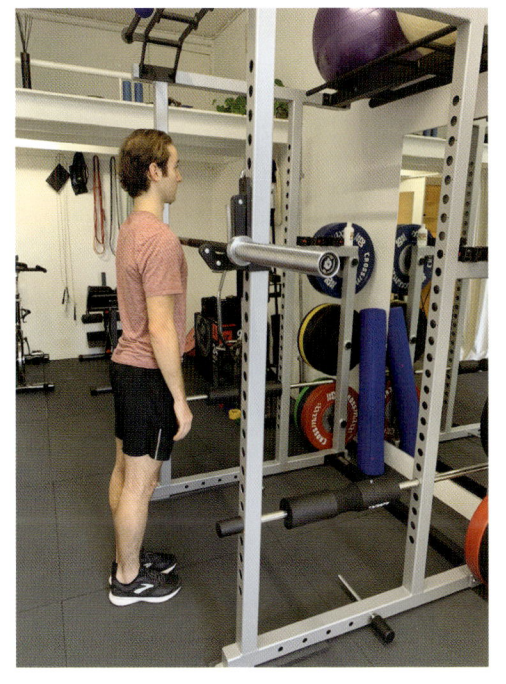

Fig. 97 Front squat set-up.

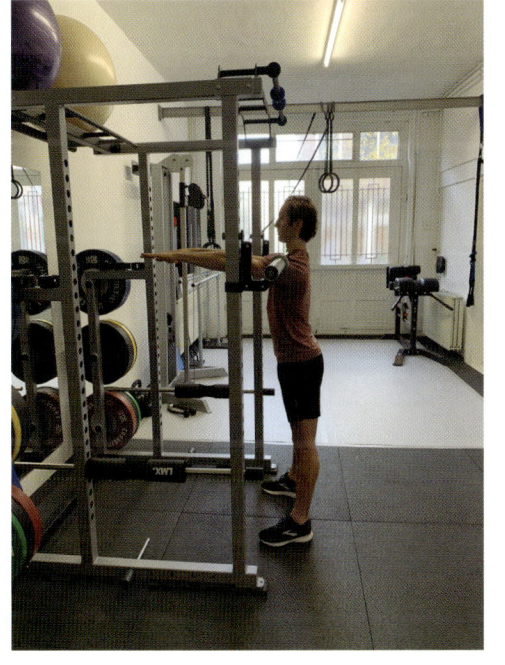

Fig. 98 Arm position.

Fig. 99 Zombie arms.

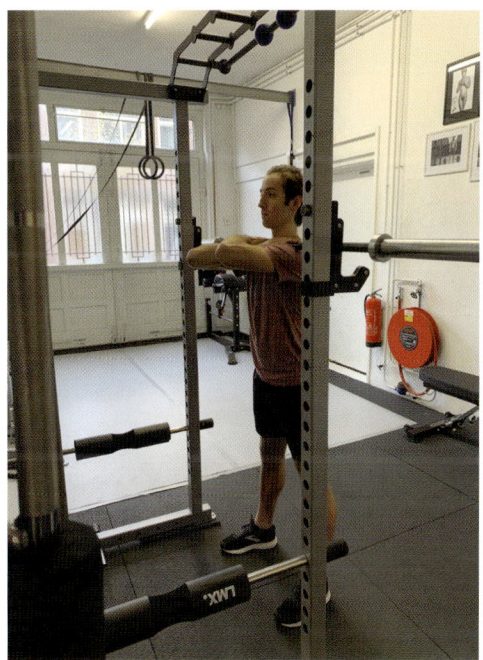

Fig. 100 Crossed arms.

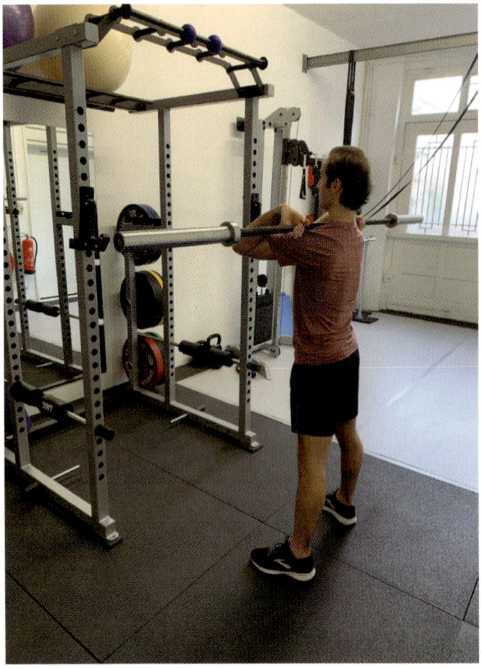

LOWER-BODY EXERCISES

Fig. 101 Front squat start position.

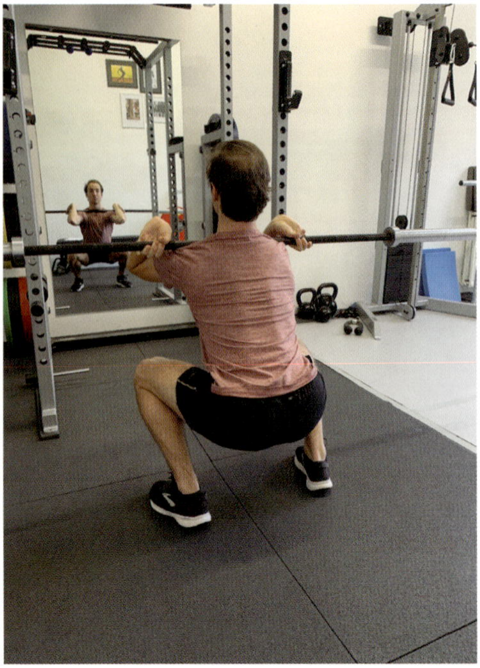

Fig. 102 Mid-movement.

Overhead squat

The overhead squat is a true test of strength and stability. It is a full-bodied exercise as everything must work in unison in order to perform it. In dance there is a lot of overhead lifting and this exercise helps to build strength and confidence in this area.

1. Begin with the pins of the squat rack set at the correct height for bar placement. This should be the same as your front squat position.
2. Get into your position by stepping under the bar, squeeze your shoulder blades together and place the bar on the ledge that has been created by this movement (Fig. 103).
3. Stand up straight so that the bar comes up and away from the pins, then take a large step back (Fig. 104).
4. Bend at the legs and in a push-press movement raise the bar overhead until your arms are locked and in-line with your ears (Fig. 105).
5. Take a big breath and brace your core.
6. Your feet should be hip- or shoulder-width apart (this should feel comfortable for you), and your feet slightly turned out.
7. Break at the knees and push your hips back as you descend.
8. Once you have reached the depth that is correct for you (Fig. 106), drive back up through the whole foot and squeeze your glutes, while letting your breath out through pursed lips (this is known as a partial Valsalva manoeuvre and helps to maintain your brace throughout the exercise).
9. Once you have reached the top, take another breath and repeat the whole process.
10. When you have completed the required number of repetitions, lower the bar onto your back as it was in the beginning and then re-rack the bar.

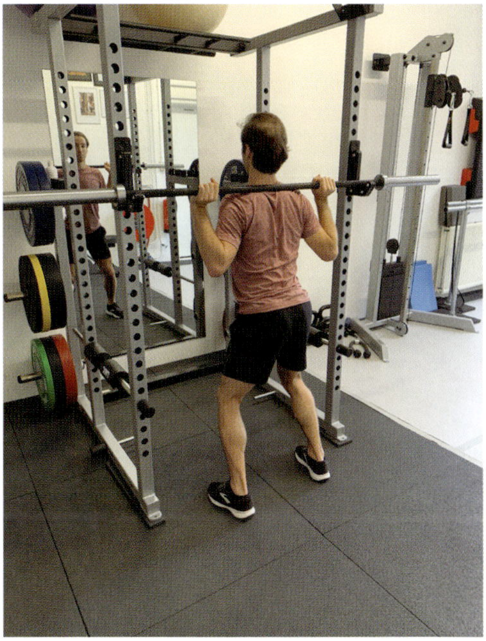

LOWER-BODY EXERCISES

Fig. 103 Overhead squat set-up.

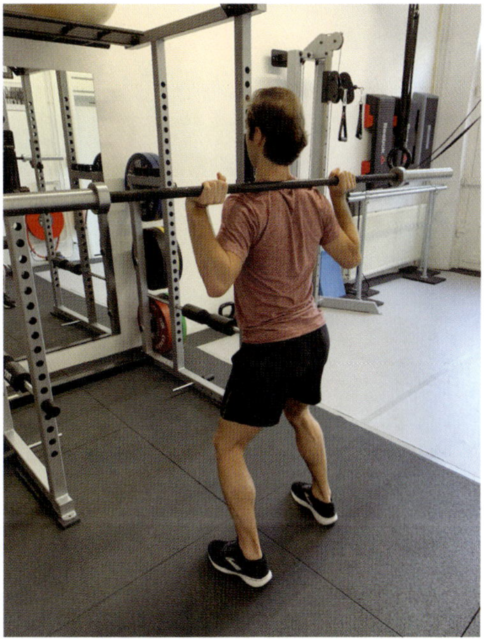

Fig. 104 Initial start position.

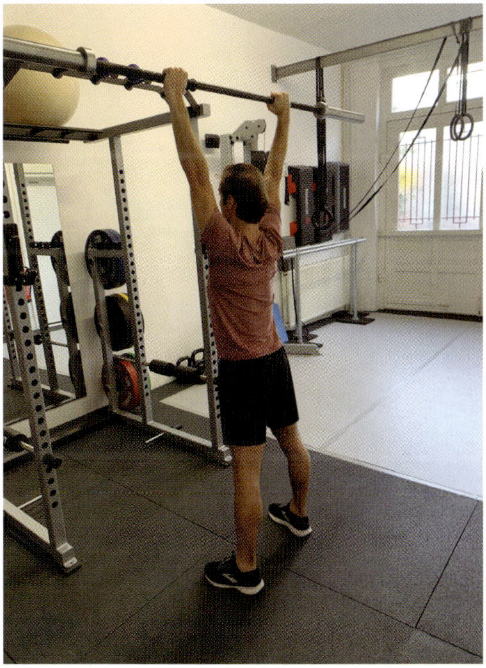

Fig. 105 Start position.

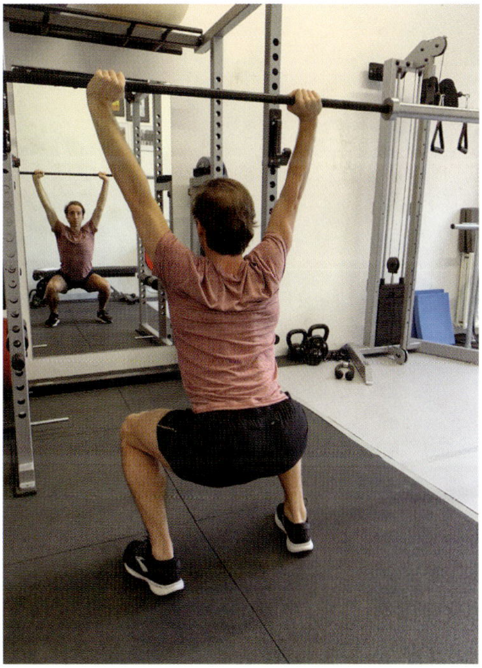

Fig. 106 Mid-movement.

LOWER-BODY EXERCISES

Unilateral and Bilateral Hip Dominant

Glute bridges

The glute bridge is a good way to introduce hip hingeing. It helps to strengthen the glutes and hamstrings and can be made harder by adding a barbell across the hips. You can also perform these as a single-leg exercise, which is harder.

1. Begin by lying supine (on your back), on the floor with your legs bent at a 90-degree angle (this can be larger if necessary); this ensures that you will be using your hamstrings and glutes with minimal quadriceps activation (Fig. 107).
2. The closer your feet are to your bottom the more you will recruit the quadriceps.
3. Squeeze your glutes and raise your hips from the floor until you have reached full extension (Fig. 108).
4. Be careful not to overarch with this as you will feel it in your lower back.
5. Lower your hips until you reach the ground and repeat for the required number of repetitions.
6. Figs 109 and 110 show a single-leg version.

*Note: to increase gluteus medius activation you can add a small band just below the knees.

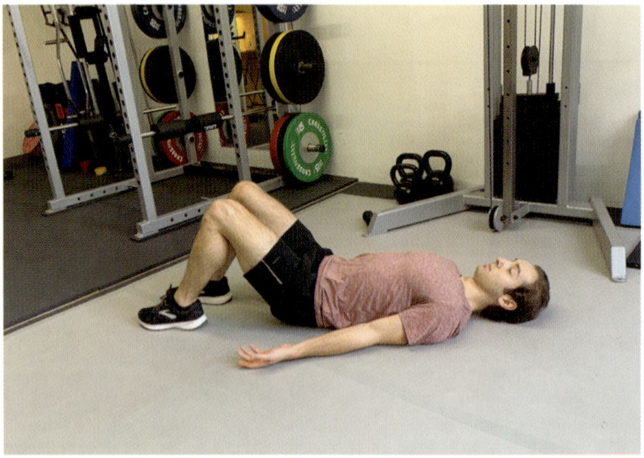

Fig. 107 Overhead squat set-up.

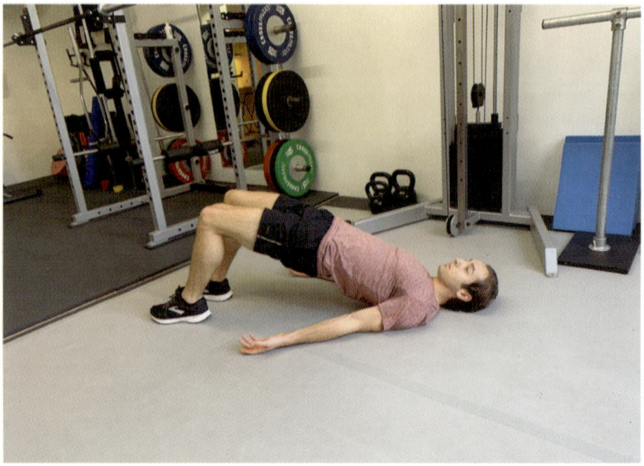

Fig. 108 Initial start position.

LOWER-BODY EXERCISES

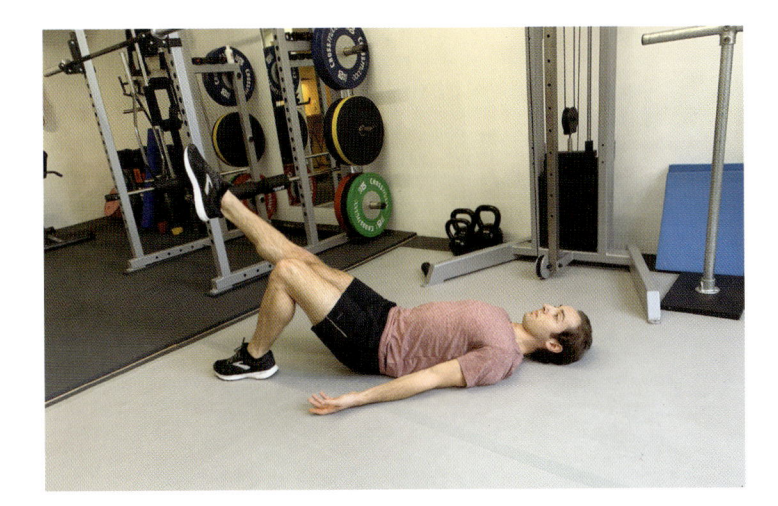

Fig. 109 Start position.

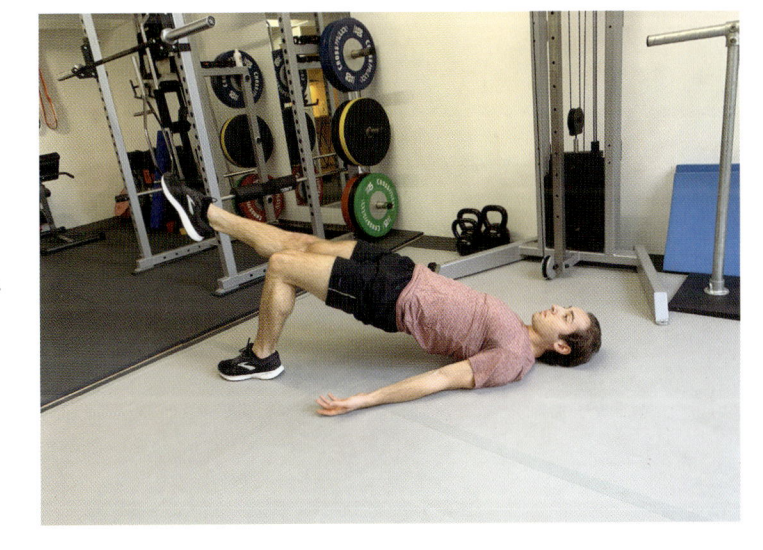

Fig. 110 Mid-movement.

Hip thrusts

The only difference between a glute bridge and a hip thrust is that the back is placed on a higher surface to increase the range of motion. This can be anything from a low step to a bench. In order to add load to this you can place a barbell across your hips with a pad in place. You can also perform these as single-leg exercises to make them harder.

1. Begin by placing your upper back just below your shoulder blades on the step/ bench, bent at a 90-degree angle (this can be larger if necessary); this ensures that you will be using your hamstrings and glutes with minimal quadriceps activation (Fig. 111).
2. The closer your feet are to your bottom the more you will recruit the quadriceps.
3. Squeezing your glutes raise your hips from the floor until you have reached full extension (Fig. 112).
4. Be careful not to overarch with this, as you will feel it in your lower back. Lower your hips until you reach the ground.
5. Repeat for the required number of repetitions.

105

LOWER-BODY EXERCISES

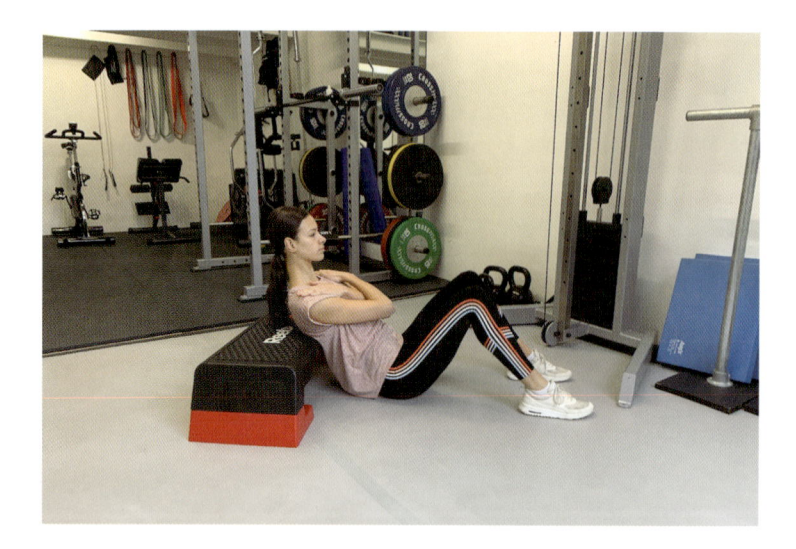

Fig. 111
Hip thrust start position.

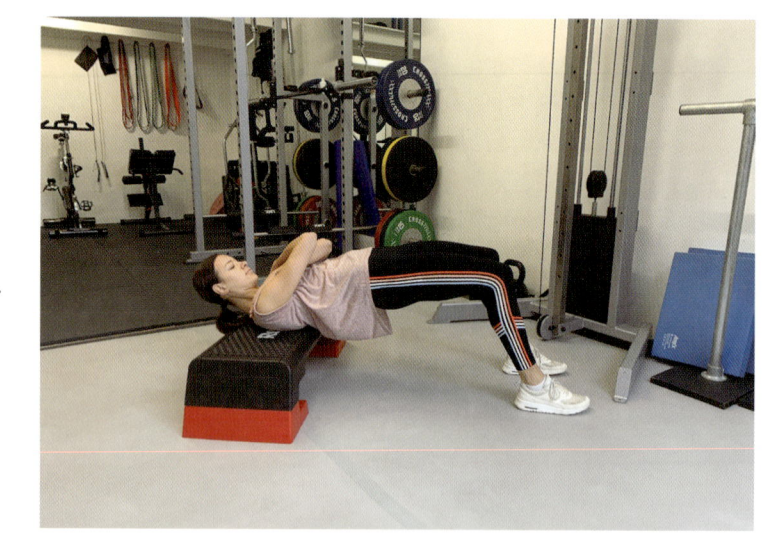

Fig. 112
Mid-movement.

Single leg single arm deadlift

This works not only as a hip hinge exercise – it also has an anti-rotational aspect to it. This can be performed with opposing legs and arms or on the same side. In this version we are using a kettlebell to perform it.

1. Begin with the kettlebell in your hand and placed at your side (Fig. 113).
2. Brace your core.
3. Then moving your hips backward and your leg in the air of the opposing side, lower the kettlebell to the ground, making sure to keep a neutral spine (Fig. 114).
4. Squeeze your glutes to begin bringing your leg down and hips back to the beginning position.
5. The movement should only be at your hips.
6. Repeat for the required number of repetitions.

LOWER-BODY EXERCISES

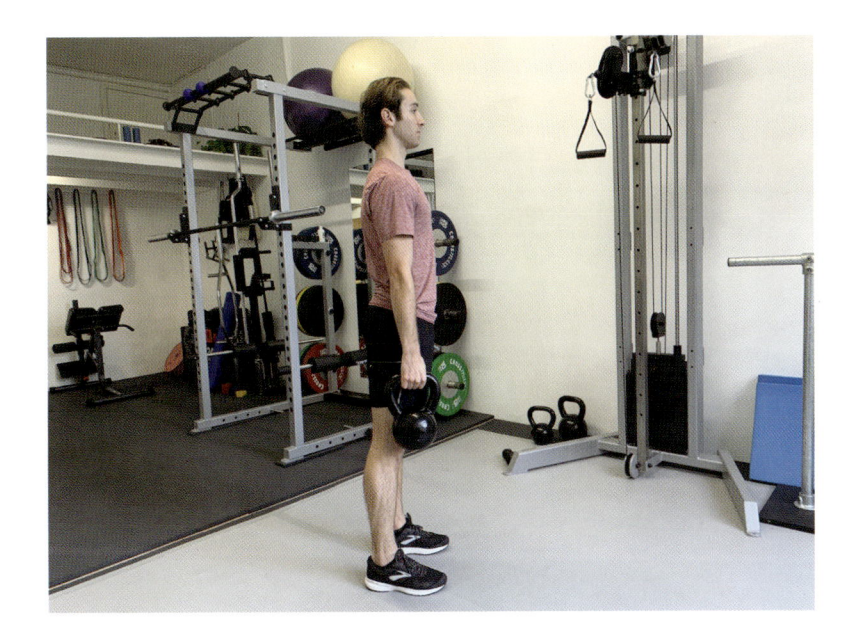

Fig. 113
Single leg single arm deadlift start position.

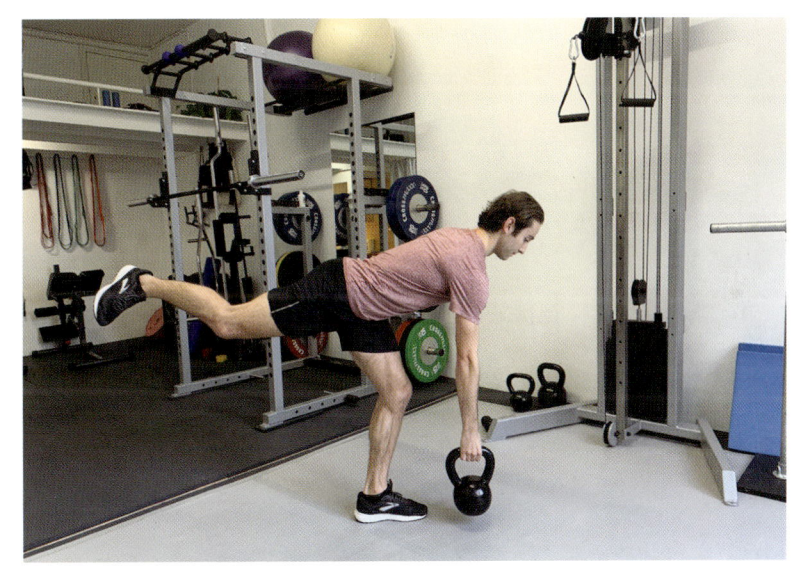

Fig. 114
Mid-movement.

Reverse hyper-extensions

This exercise is a fantastic way to introduce posterior chain training in a safe and effective manner. Due to the nature of this movement, it also has a decompressive effect on the spine while being performed. There are many, many ways to do this exercise and it can be graded simply by moving the hips closer to or further away from the fulcrum of the machine being used. This movement is also a nice way of introducing a hip hinge. It trains the erectors, glutes and hamstrings. These exercises can be

107

LOWER-BODY EXERCISES

performed with a single leg as a regression for the glutes and hamstrings while acting as an endurance exercise for the low back.

Place the machine in the correct position for your needs: the closer your hips are to the fulcrum of the pads of the machine, the easier it becomes and the less your erectors and glutes have to work.

1. Put your hands on the handles and slide yourself into position. Your legs should be hanging down over the pad (Fig. 115).
2. Raise both legs up keeping them as straight as possible until they are parallel to the ground and externally rotate from the hips a little to engage the glutes more (Fig. 116).
3. Once in the top position, lower your legs until they are at the beginning point.
4. Repeat for the required repetitions.
5. There should be minimal movement from the spine.

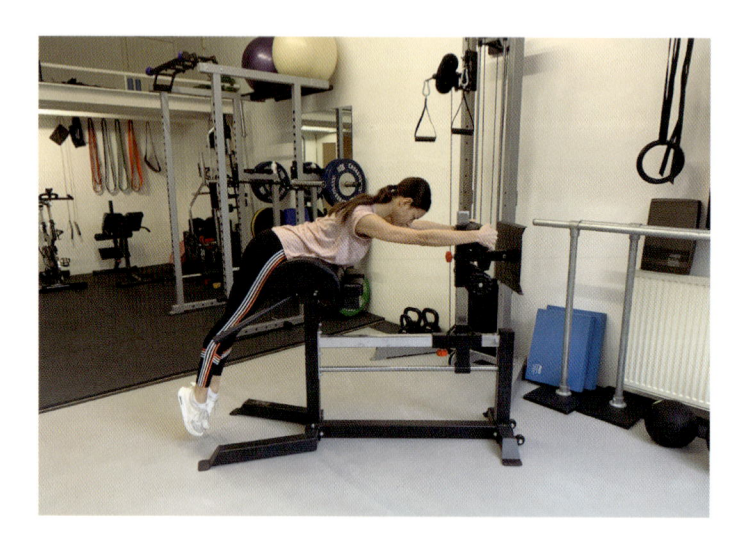

Fig. 115 Reverse hyper-extension start position.

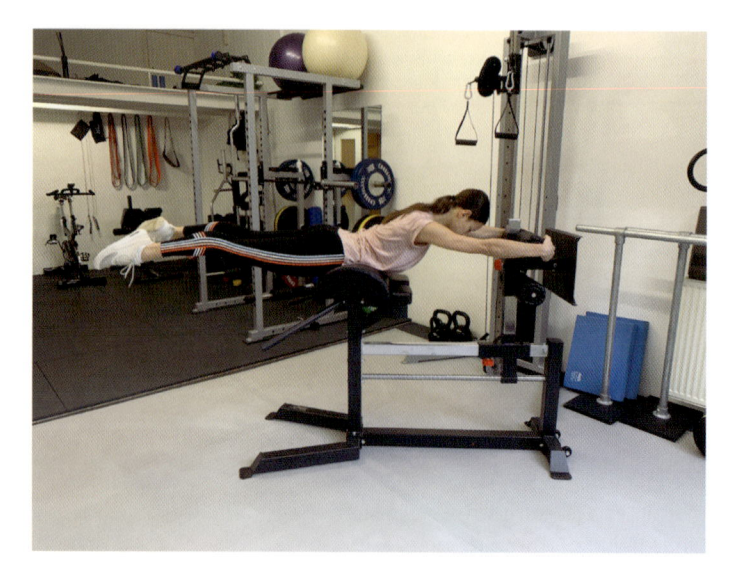

Fig. 116 Mid-movement.

LOWER-BODY EXERCISES

45-degree back extension

Much like the reverse hyper, this exercise is great to help with the hip hinge movement and can be made easier or harder depending on where the hips are placed around the pads of the machine. It trains the erectors, glutes and hamstrings. The single-leg version of these is very advanced and requires a good amount of strength to perform it.

1. Place the machine in the correct position for your level. The further over the pads your hips are, the more difficult the exercise becomes.
2. Once you have placed your feet between the foot pads and positioned yourself over the machine (Fig. 117), lower your upper body as far down as possible without rounding the lower back.
3. Once in this bottom position contract your glutes and bring your body up until it is at your beginning position (Fig. 118).
4. Be careful not to over-extend the back.
5. Repeat for the desired repetitions.

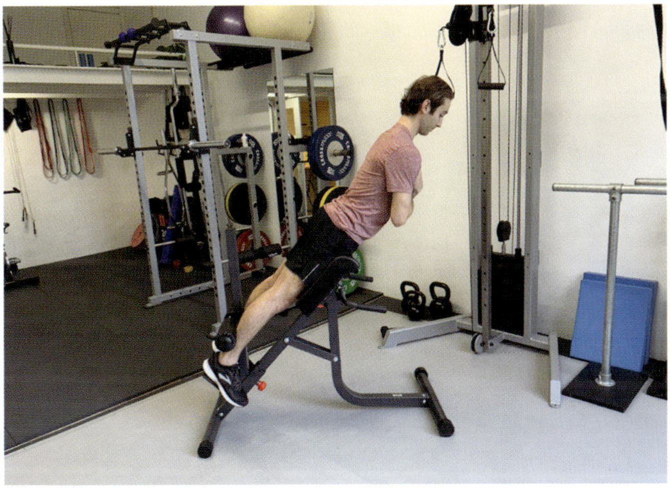

Fig. 117 45-degree back extension start position.

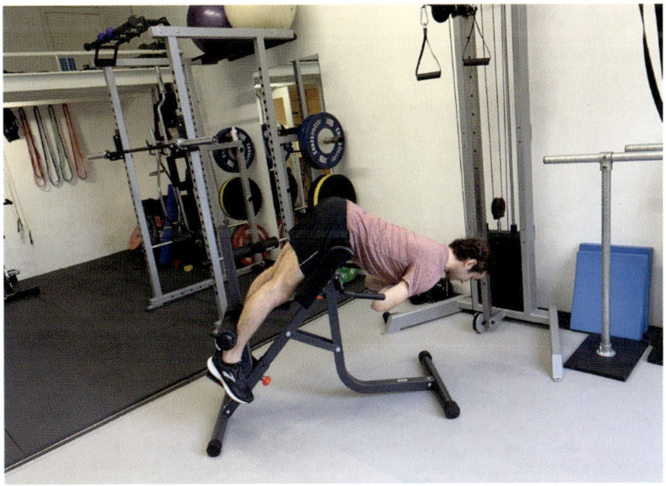

Fig. 118 Mid-movement.

LOWER-BODY EXERCISES

Back extension

The back extension is a slightly more difficult version of the 45-degree one due to the setup of the machine and the line of pull. The single-leg version of these is very advanced and requires a good amount of strength to perform it.

1. Place the machine in the correct position for your level. The further over the pads your hips are, the more difficult the exercise becomes.
2. Once you have placed your feet between the foot pads and positioned yourself over the machine, lower your upper body as far down as possible.
3. Once in this position, begin by finding a good straight back (Fig. 119).
4. Start the movement by contracting your glutes and bringing your body up until it is parallel to the ground (Fig. 120), being careful not to over-extend the back.
5. Once in the top position, move from the hips once again to lower the upper body into the starting point, making sure there is minimum movement of the spine.
6. Repeat for the desired repetitions.

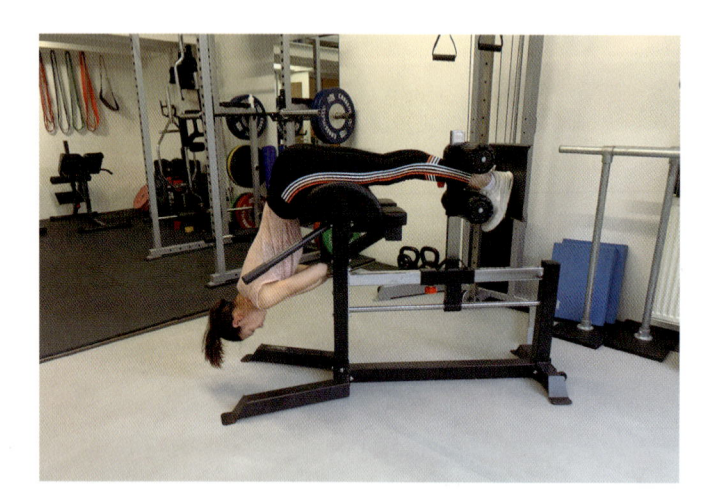

Fig. 119
Back extension start position.

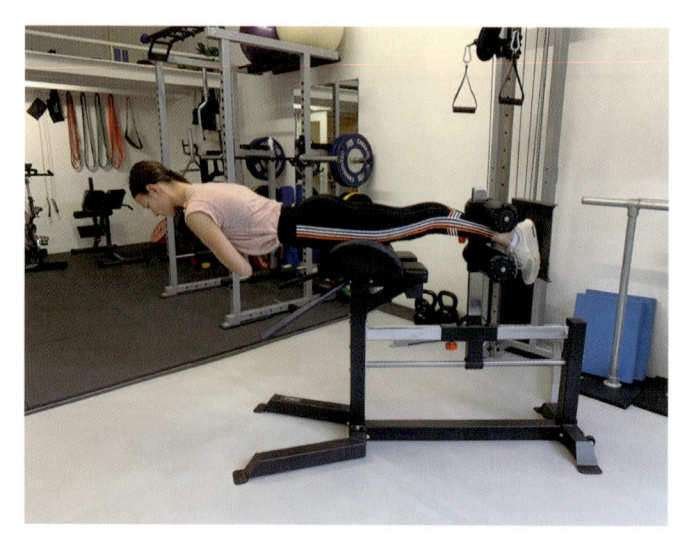

Fig. 120
Mid-movement.

LOWER-BODY EXERCISES

Rack pull

This exercise works the erectors, glutes and hamstrings. It is a great exercise for both the beginner and the advanced trainee. For the beginner it can be good to help teach the hip hinge in a standing position and for the advanced to help with the top or lockout position of the deadlift.

1. Set the pins in the squat rack to just below the knees.
2. When everything is set, step towards the bar until the shins are touching the bar.
3. Push your hips back as you lower your body to take the bar in your hands, with your legs slightly bent.
4. Pull the bar against your shins to lock your lats in place (Fig. 121).
5. Take a breath and create a brace.
6. Contract your glutes hard as you pull the bar from the pins and raise it until you are standing tall (Fig. 122).
7. Make sure to continue to contract your glutes in the top position and imagine that you want to bend the bar around your hips as this will keep tension in your lats when you have reached lockout.
8. When lowering the bar, push the hips back and break at the knees very slightly while keeping the bar against your legs.
9. Once the bar has travelled past your knees bend them until the bar is resting against the pins.
10. Remember to let your breath out through pursed lips as you lower the bar.
11. Take another breath and repeat the movement for the desired number of repetitions.

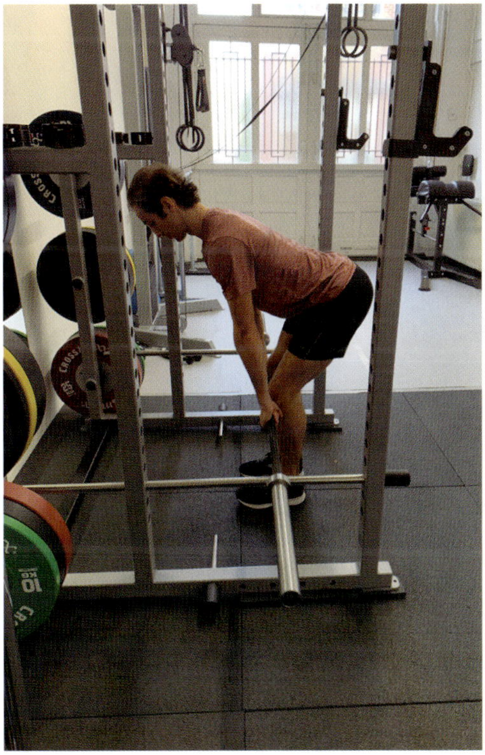

Fig. 121 Rack pull start position.

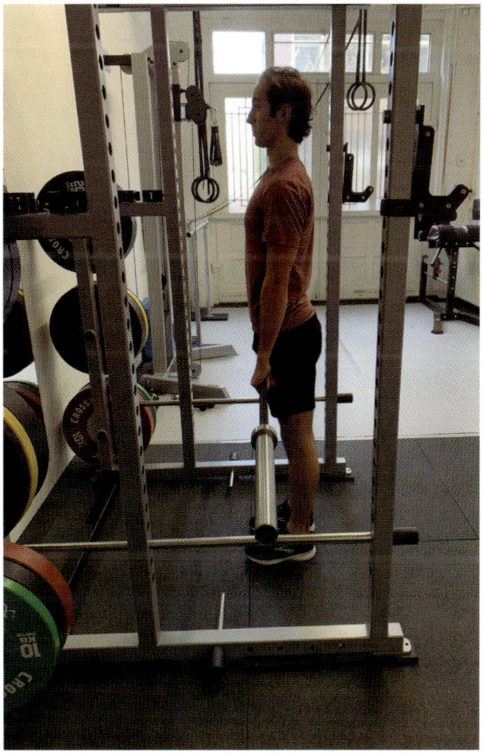

Fig. 122 Mid-movement.

LOWER-BODY EXERCISES

Trap bar deadlift

The difference between the trap bar squat and deadlift is in the positioning of the hips. When the hips are lower down the knees will have to bend more, which in turn makes it a more knee-dominant movement. When the hips are higher the movement will come from the hips to a much larger degree (hip-dominant movement). This variation of the deadlift focuses on the hamstrings, glutes and erectors; however, it is very much a full-bodied exercise. The spine is in a more stacked position due to the position of the handles being by the side which decreases shearing forces on the spine.

1. Stand inside the trap bar with your feet hip- or shoulder-width apart (this should feel comfortable for you), your feet should also be in a comfortable position and there can be some turn out from them.
2. Bend down and take the handles on either side.
3. Straighten up your back and push your hips up in the air.
4. Lock your lats by pulling up against the handles but not actually lifting the weight. Imagine that you are pulling the bar behind you a little.
5. You should now be in your deadlift position (Fig. 123).
6. Take a breath and brace your core.
7. Drive up through the whole foot and squeeze your glutes.
8. Once at the top (the top position is the same as that of the trap-bar squat), you can either take another breath or continue to hold as you lower the bar back down to the ground.
9. Repeat the process for the required number of repetitions.

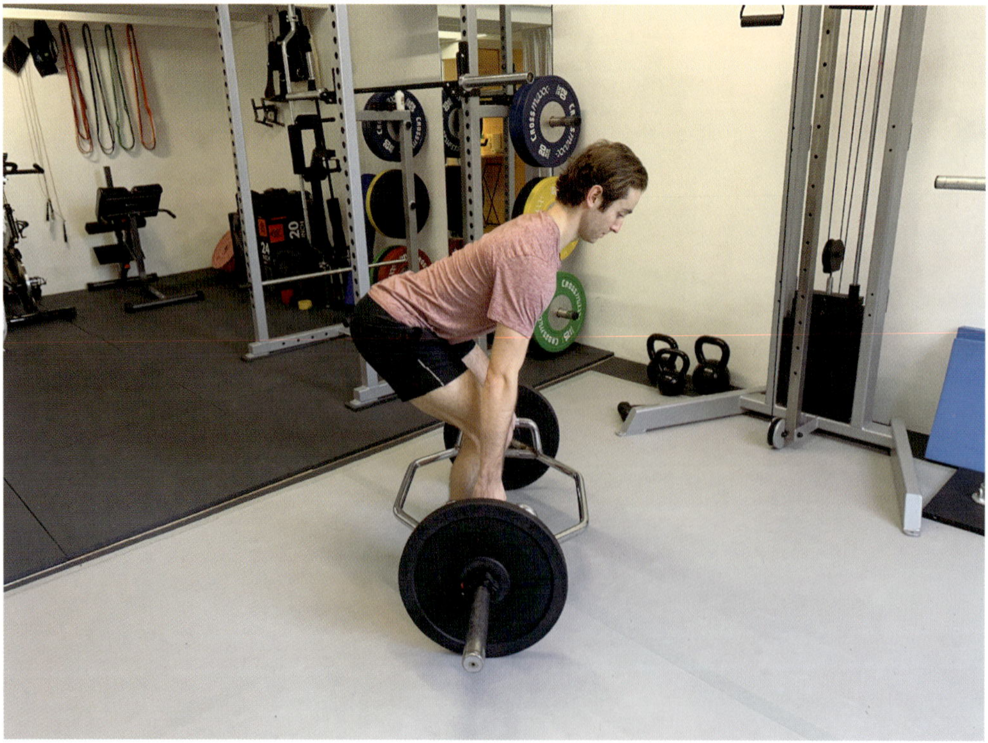

Fig. 123 Trap bar deadlift mid-movement.

LOWER-BODY EXERCISES

Staggered stance deadlift

The staggered stance version of this makes it slightly more unilateral. The set-up is exactly the same as the trap bar deadlift except that you place one foot slightly behind you in a very small split stance. There should be roughly a 70:30 split in terms of weight distribution.

1. Stand inside the trap bar with your feet hip- or shoulder-width apart, as explained in the trap bar deadlift.
2. Bend down and take the handles on either side, straighten up your back and push your hips up in the air.
3. Lock your lats by pulling up against the handles but not actually lifting the weight.
4. Imagine also that you are pulling the bar behind you a little. You should now be in your deadlift position (Fig. 124).
5. Take a breath and brace your core.
6. Drive up through the whole foot, squeezing your glutes until you arrive in the top position (Fig. 125).
7. Once at the top you can either take another breath or continue to hold as you lower the bar back down to the ground.
8. Repeat the process for the required number of repetitions.

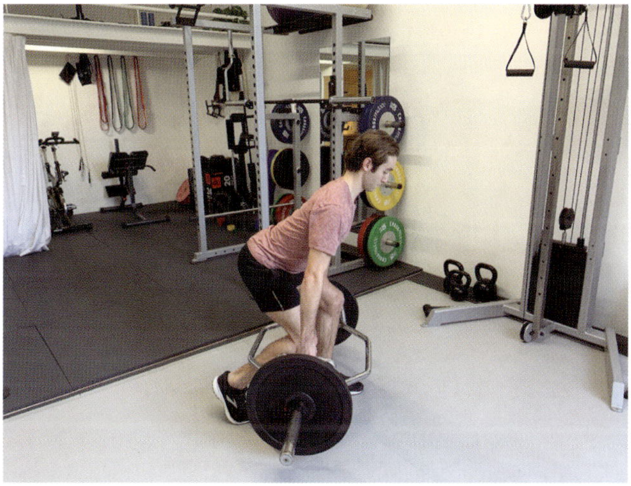

Fig. 124 Staggered stance deadlift start position.

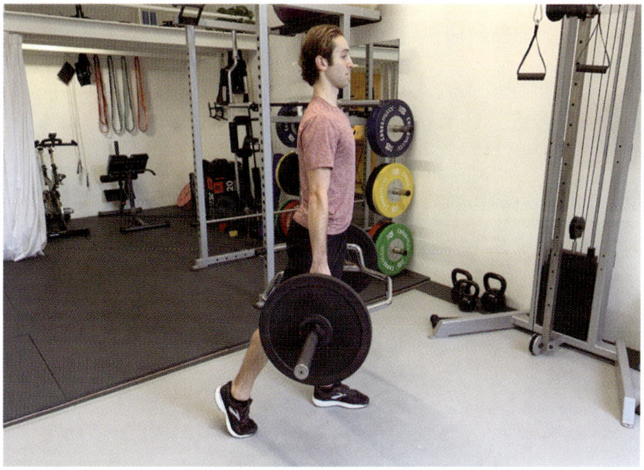

Fig. 125 Mid-movement.

LOWER-BODY EXERCISES

Sumo deadlift

This exercise works the adductors to a much greater degree than other deadlift variations. It is also more spine friendly, in that you can be in a more upright position. The focus is on the posterior chain but again it is a full-bodied exercise due to the number of secondary muscles used.

1. Stand with your feet in a wide position; this can be shoulder width or wider depending on your anatomy.
2. Your toes should be pointing outwards with the knees still tracking over the second toe.
3. The toes should be showing on the other side of the barbell.
4. Break at the hips first, then the knees as you go down to grab the bar.
5. Your hands should be on the outside of your shins, chest should be high, and chin tucked.
6. Create some tension against the bar before you lift by gripping it hard and pulling against it (Fig. 126).
7. Take a big breath and brace just before you begin to lift.
8. As you begin to pull the bar from the ground, think of the cue, 'push the floor away'.
9. The first part of the lift will be mainly leg dominant and as the bar clears the knees the hips will play the greater role.
10. Keep squeezing your glutes as you drive the bar against your hips to complete the lift (Fig. 127).
11. Once at the top you can either take another breath or continue to hold as you lower the bar.
12. When lowering the bar, break at the hips and push them back while very slightly bending at the knee, making sure to keep the bar against your legs. This part of the lift is mainly from your hips.
13. Once the bar has travelled past your knees, bend them until the bar touches the ground.
14. Repeat for the required number of repetitions.

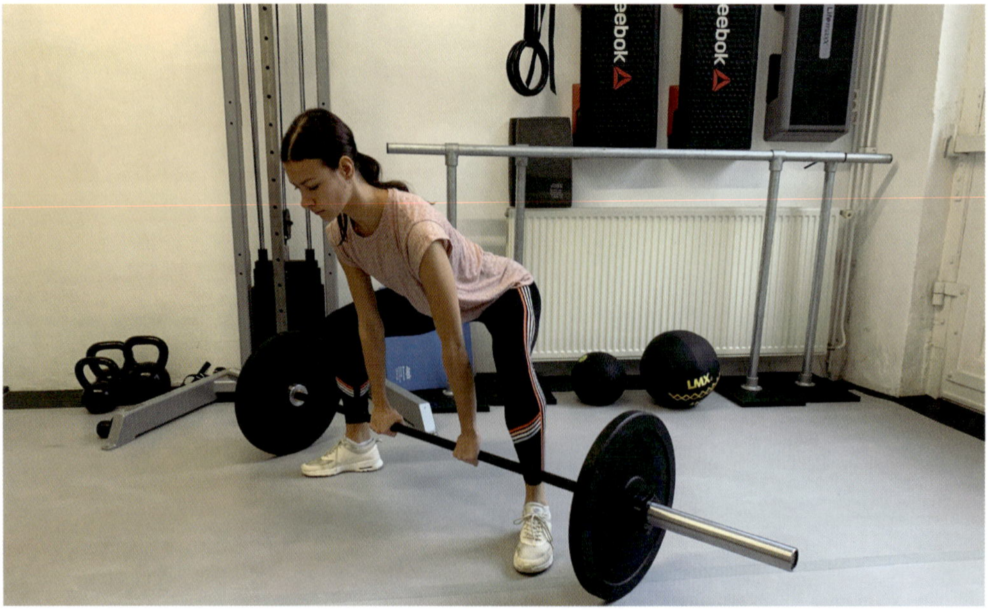

Fig. 126 Sumo squat start position.

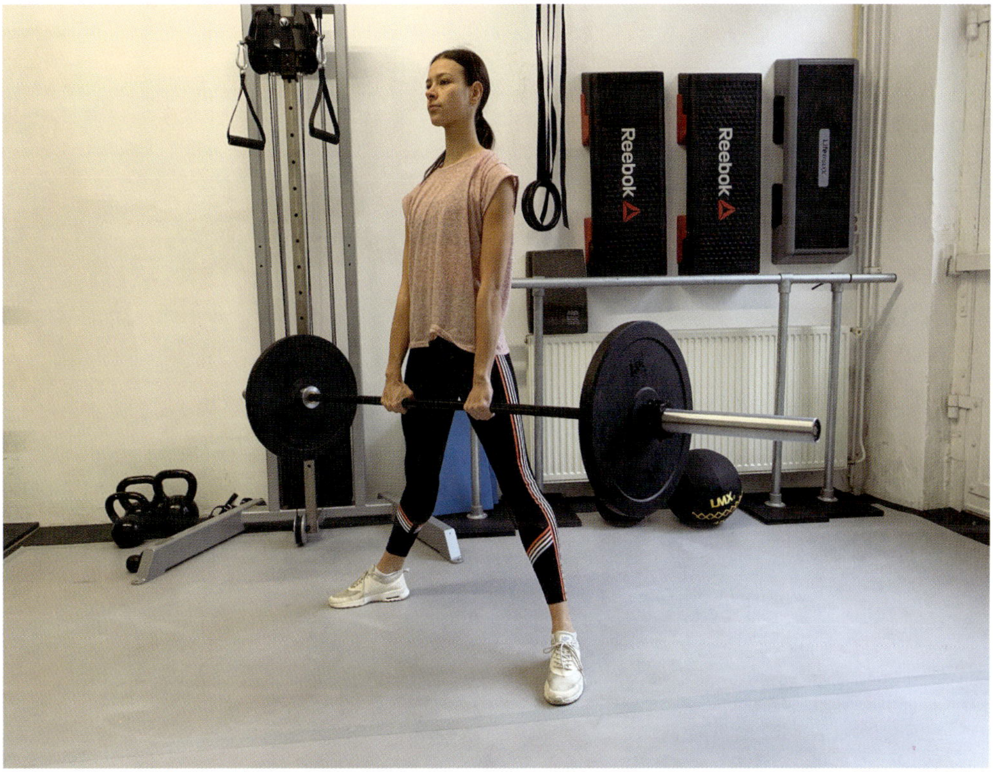

LOWER-BODY EXERCISES

Fig. 127 Mid-movement.

KNEE FLEXION EXERCISES

The hamstrings have two main functions: hip extension and knee flexion. The hip hingeing exercises take care of the former while these exercises address the latter.

Stability ball hamstring curls

With this exercise you start to incorporate the posterior chain a little more and there is a stability component to it.

1. Place your feet on the ball slightly apart from each other; the more of the ball that covers your legs the easier the exercise is.
2. Put your hands out to the side with your palms facing upwards, this ensures that you keep your shoulders from rising up (Fig. 128).
3. Raise your hips off the ground (Fig. 129) and roll the ball towards your glutes, keeping the hips as high as possible but without over-arching (Fig. 130).
4. Roll the ball out to the beginning position.
5. Repeat for the required number of repetitions.

To make this harder for stability purposes you can bring the arms in towards the body. To make the exercise harder on the hamstrings you can do the single-leg version (Fig. 131).

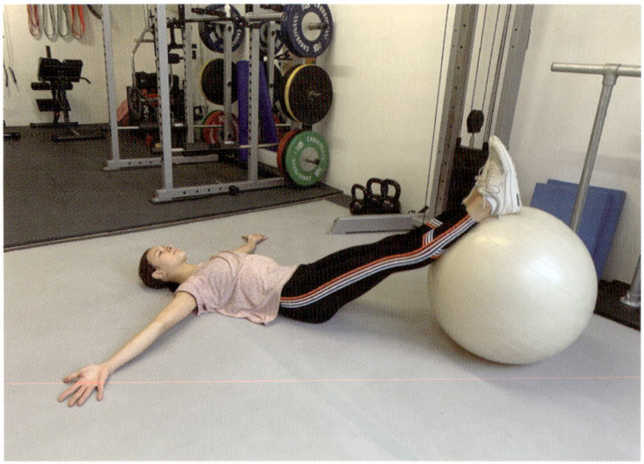

LOWER-BODY EXERCISES

Fig. 128 Stability ball hamstring curls set-position.

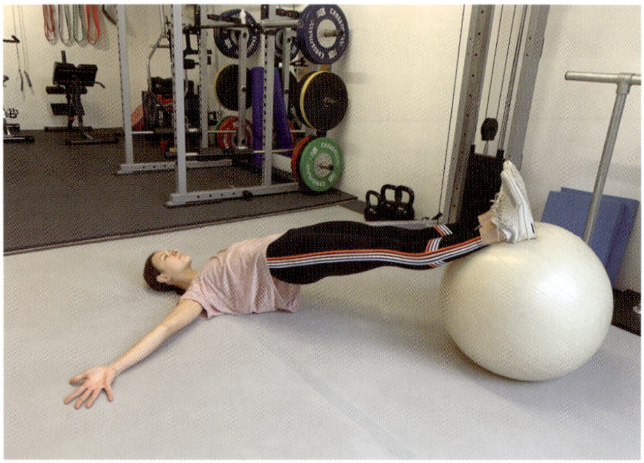

Fig. 129 Start position.

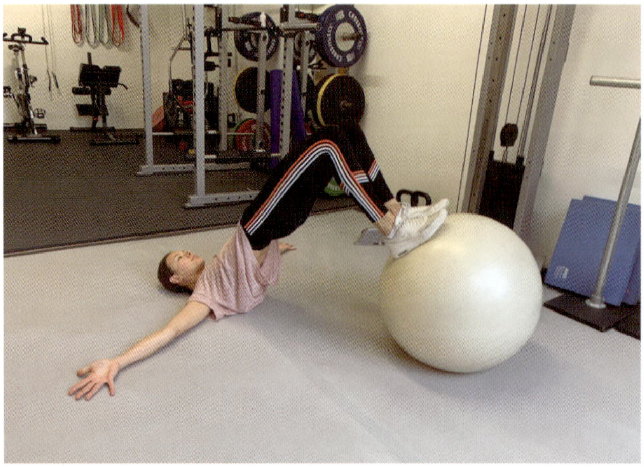

Fig. 130 Mid-movement.

LOWER-BODY EXERCISES

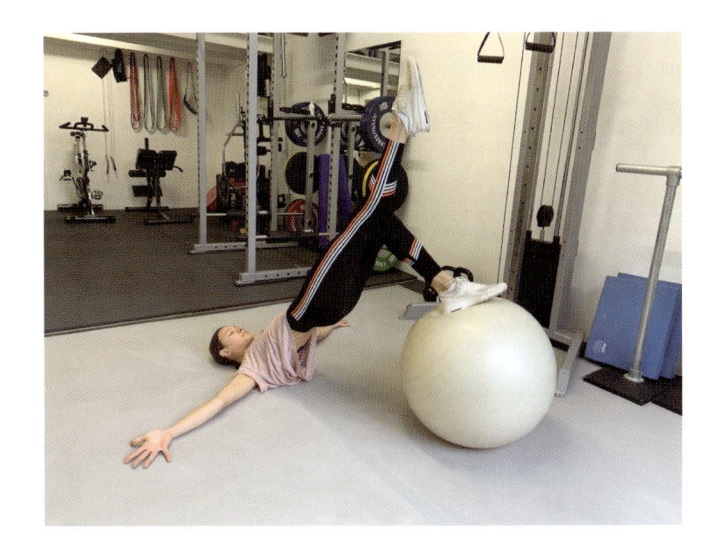

Fig. 131
Advanced version.

Floor slide hamstring curls

This is a deceptively difficult exercise to perform and thus is seen as a more advanced version of the stability ball hamstring curl. Depending on the surface you may need something in order to make sure that you can slide your feet back and forth across the floor.

1. Place yourself supine (on your back) on the ground and bend your legs so that they are as close to your glutes as possible.
2. Place your hands out to the side with your palms facing down (Fig. 132).
3. Raise your hips off the ground (Fig. 133) and slide your feet away until you reach end range (Fig. 134).
4. Begin to bring them back in, all the while trying to keep your hips high.
5. Repeat for the required number of repetitions.

To make this even more challenging you can try the single-leg version (Figs 135 and 136).

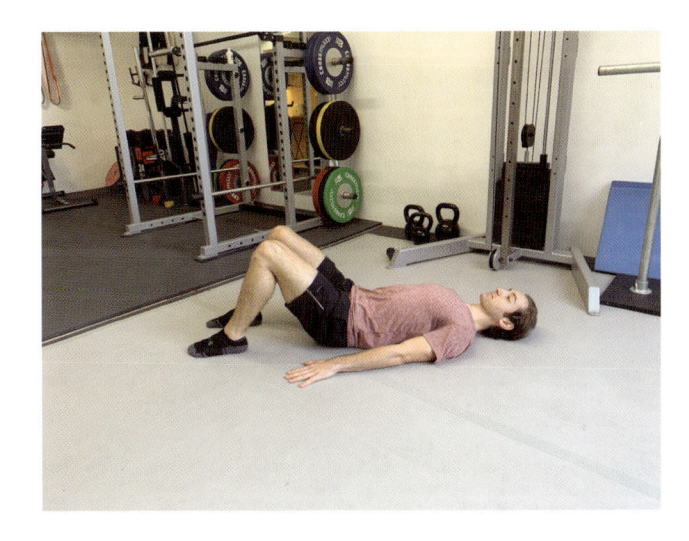

Fig. 132 Floor slide hamstring curl set-up position.

117

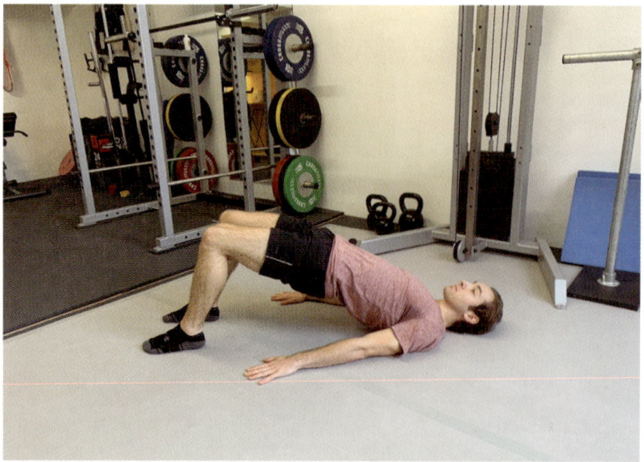

LOWER-BODY EXERCISES

Fig. 133 Start position.

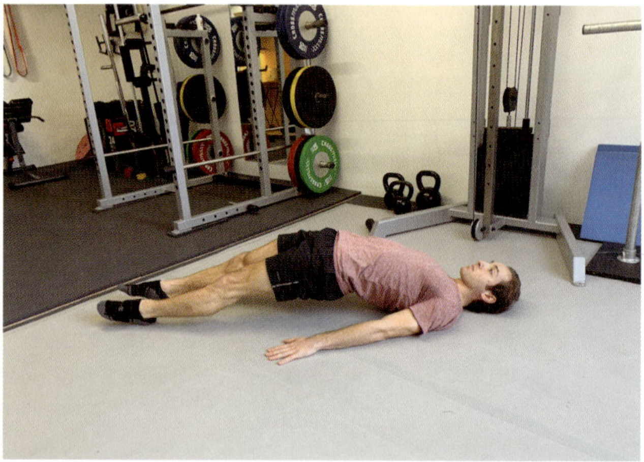

Fig. 134 Mid-movement.

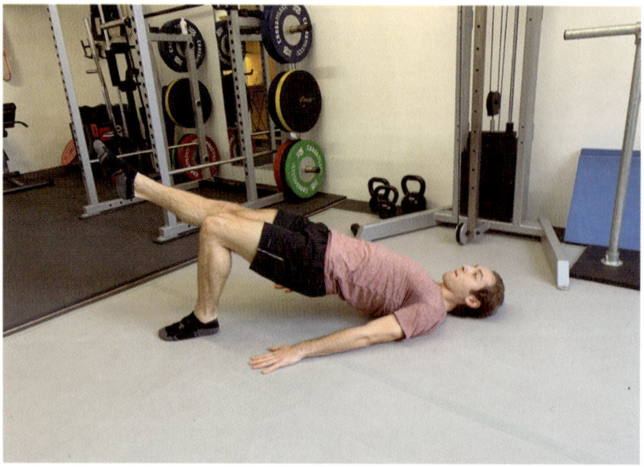

Fig. 135 Advanced start position.

118

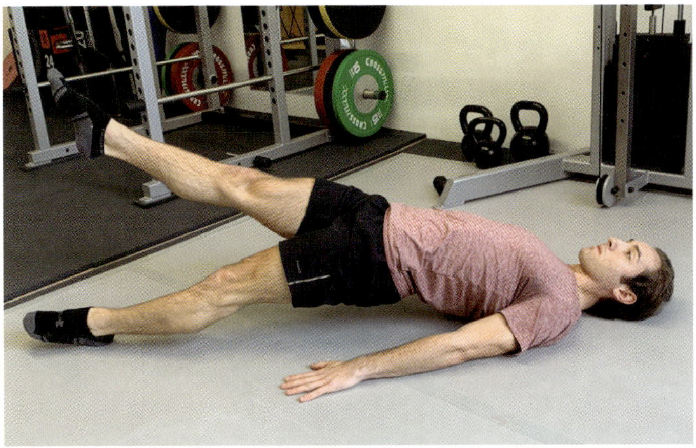

LOWER-BODY EXERCISES

Fig. 136 Advanced mid-position.

Glute ham raises

The glute ham raise is one the best knee flexion exercises that you can do and there are many variations for this one exercise. In this variation we will focus on the simplest one.

1. Make sure to set the machine to the correct position for you, so that your hips are just over the fulcrum of the pad.
2. Start in an upright position with your arms across your chest (Fig. 137).
3. Slowly lower yourself downwards (Fig. 138) so that your arms are touching the pad (this is your start and end position) and slide down until you are almost straight at the knee (Fig. 139).
4. Once in this position imagine pulling yourself backwards from the knee.
5. Once you have cleared the fulcrum of the pad, repeat the exercise for the required number of repetitions.

*Note: those deemed hyper-flexible must stay away from the end range of this exercise.

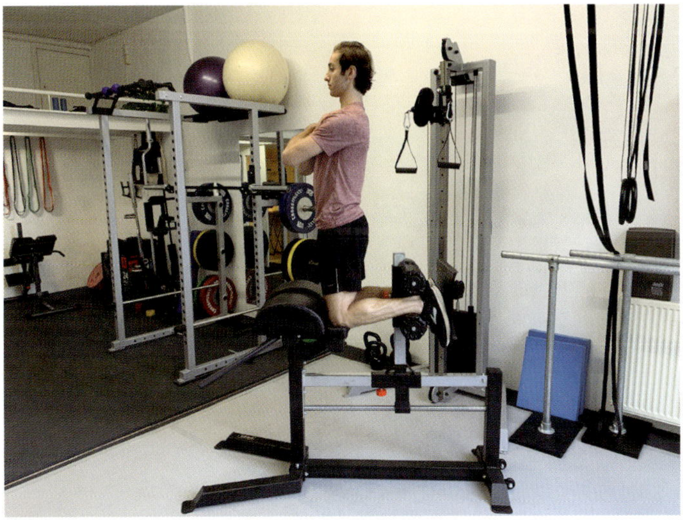

Fig. 137 Glute ham raises set-up position.

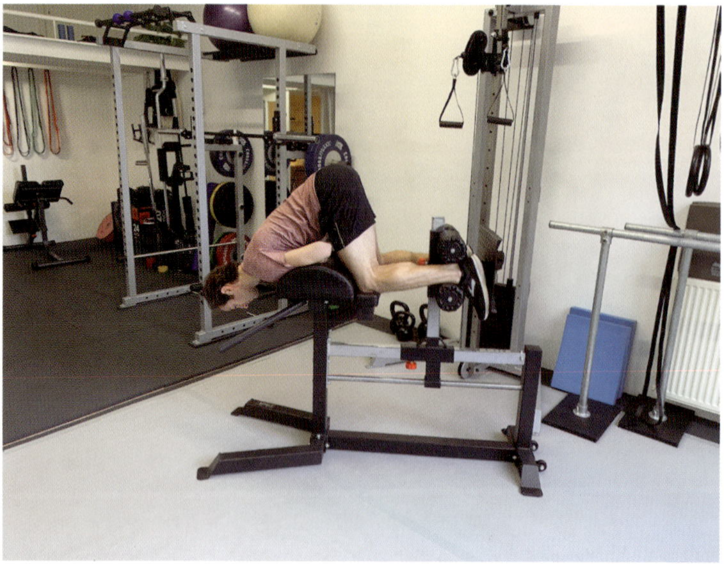

LOWER-BODY EXERCISES

Fig. 138 Start position.

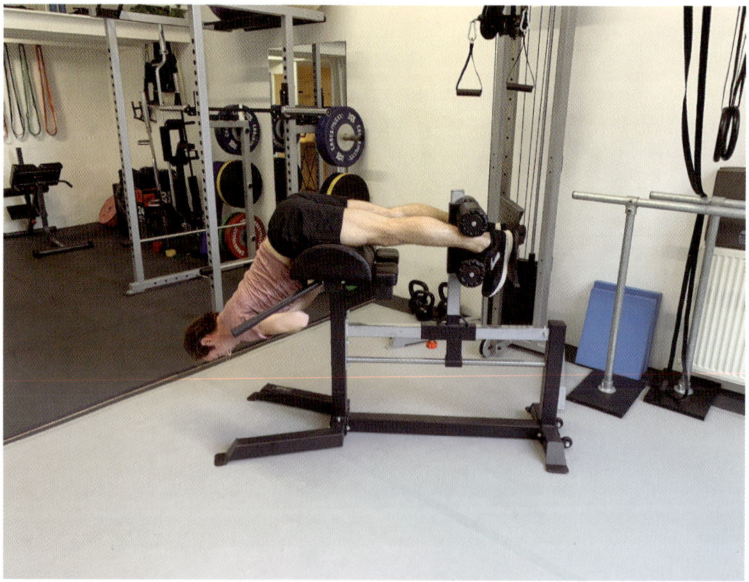

Fig. 139 Mid-movement.

8 | UPPER-BODY EXERCISES

We have included a variety of exercises that include body-resistance and resistance equipment movements for the upper body. Again, we have focused on closed-kinetic chain movements, rather than open-chain exercises such as bicep curls. This is not to exclude the latter (these are especially pertinent if there is a muscular imbalance), but we feel that closed-kinetic chain movements are more functional and engage a larger number of muscles to carry out the exercises.

BODY WEIGHT RESISTANCE

Incline push-up

The incline push-up is a great place to start when push-ups from the ground aren't yet possible. It will help to ensure that the scapulae are moving well, and the core can be maintained throughout the movement.

1. Place your hands on a bench in line with your shoulders, feet together, glutes squeezed, abdominals braced, and chin tucked.
2. You should now be in a good neutral position (Fig. 140).
3. Start to bend at the elbows and lower yourself towards the bench.
4. In the bottom position your chest must touch the bench (Fig. 141).

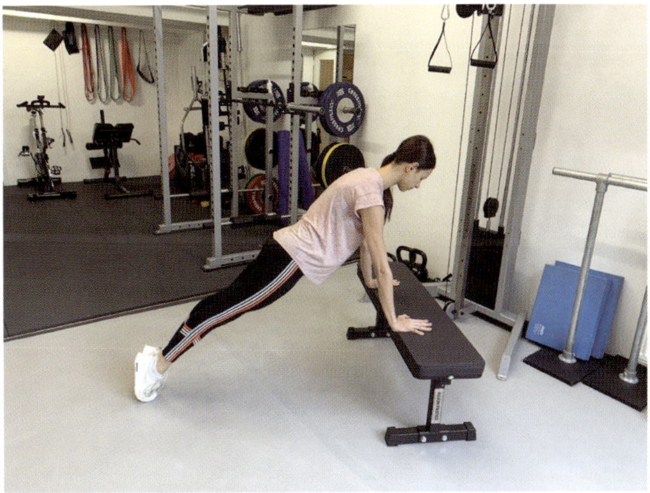

Fig. 140 Incline push-up start position.

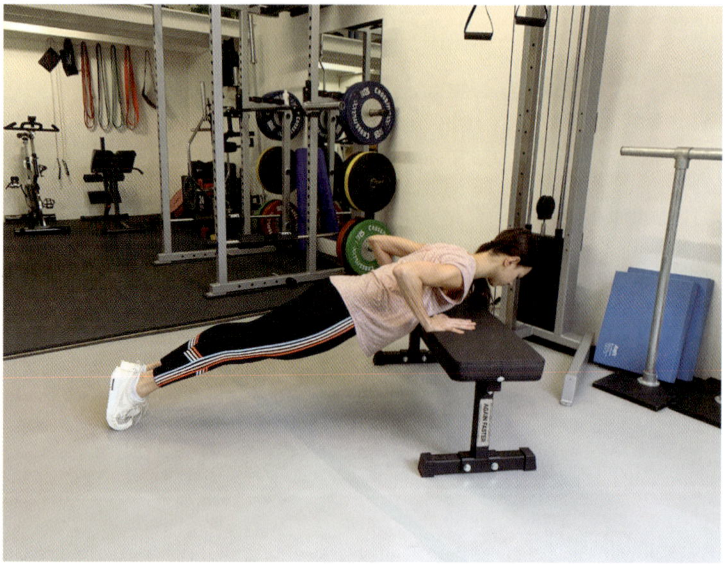

UPPER-BODY EXERCISES

Fig. 141 Mid-movement.

5. When starting to push back up, think of pushing your hands together rather than pushing yourself away.
6. Once in the top position make sure to push through your shoulder blades to activate the serratus anterior further and achieve full ROM.

Push-up

The push-up is part upper body strength work and part core work as you are in a plank position and must maintain this during the movement.

1. Start in a quadruped position: place your hands on the ground with your wrists in line with your shoulders.
2. Move your legs straight out behind you, put your feet together, squeeze your glutes, brace your abdominals gently, and tuck your chin.
3. You should now be in a good neutral position (Fig. 142).
4. To start, bend at the elbows and lower yourself towards the ground.

5. In the bottom position your chest must touch the ground.
6. Make sure to keep the whole hand in contact with the floor when starting to push up (Fig. 143), think of pushing your hands together rather than pushing yourself away.
7. Once in the top position make sure to push through your shoulder blades to activate the serratus anterior further and achieve full ROM.

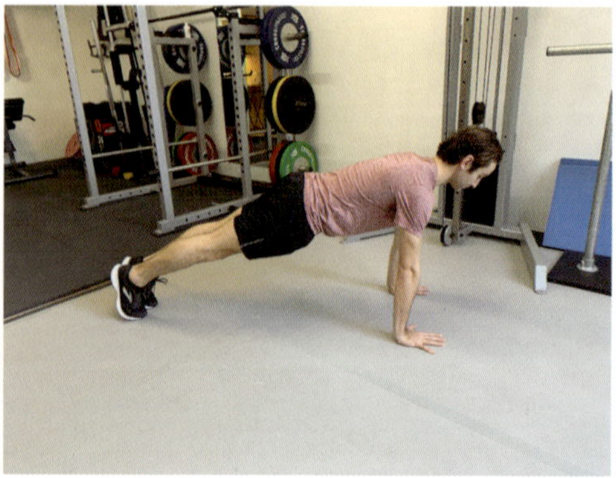

Fig. 142 Push-up start position.

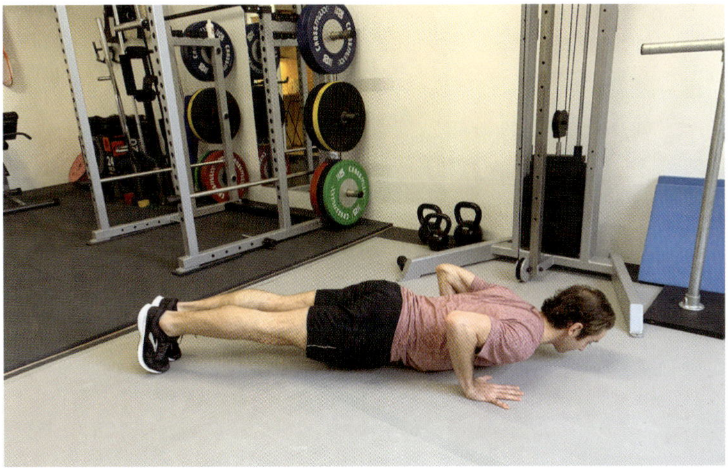

UPPER-BODY EXERCISES

Fig. 143 Mid-movement.

Decline push-up

By raising the feet, you are placing much more emphasis on the upper body, which makes it a progression from the standard push-up. Just be aware that by raising the feet you decrease the range of motion; you can place parallettes in front of you and this will resolve the issue.

1. Start in a quadruped position; place your hands on the parallettes with your wrists in line with your shoulders and move your legs straight out behind you and up onto the step which has been set at the appropriate height for you.
2. Put your feet together, squeeze your glutes, brace your abdominals gently and tuck your chin.
3. You should now be in a good neutral position (Fig. 144).
4. Start by bending at the elbows and lower yourself towards the ground.
5. Once you've reached your end range of motion (Fig. 145), begin to push up.
6. Once in the top position make sure to push through your shoulder blades to activate the serratus anterior further and achieve full ROM.
7. Repeat for the required number of repetitions.

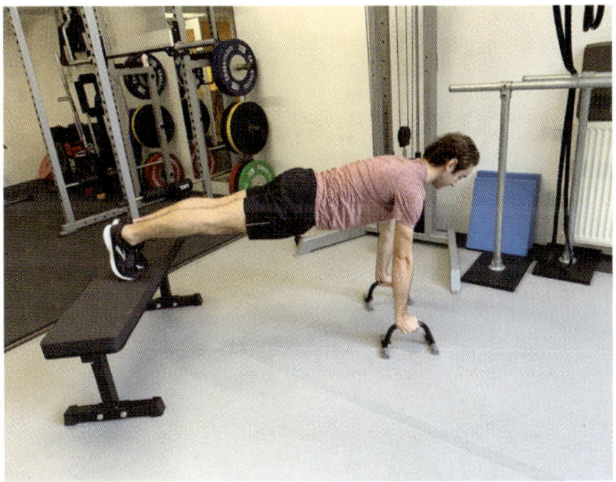

Fig. 144 Decline push-up start position.

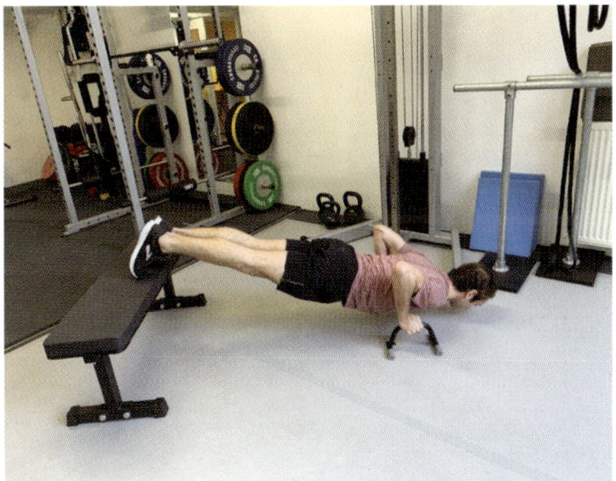

Fig. 145 Mid-movement.

UPPER-BODY EXERCISES

Pike push-ups

The pike push-up is one of the last variations of push-up before the handstand push-up. Its focus is much more on the shoulder girdle, which for dancers and overhead lifting is of the utmost importance.

1. Set a bench or box at a height where you can place your feet and bend at the hip to reach a 90-degree angle.
2. Once this has been set place your hands on the ground and your feet on the bench/box and assume a push-up position.
3. Bend at the hip until you have your head between your shoulders and your arms are in line with your ears (Fig. 146).
4. Gently lower your head towards the ground by bending your elbows until it touches the ground, then push yourself up.
5. Make sure to maintain a good brace throughout.
6. You can increase the difficulty of this by increasing the ROM with parallettes (Fig. 147).

Handstand push-ups

This exercise requires a lot of shoulder strength as well as core strength in order to maintain the position. You must also be comfortable with being able to kick up into a handstand against a wall.

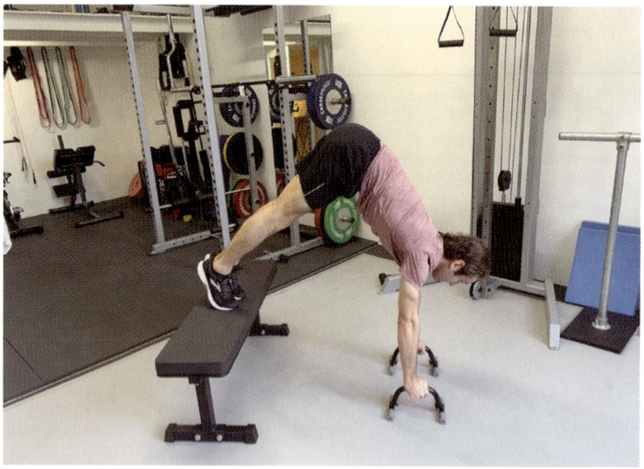

Fig. 146 Pike push-up start position.

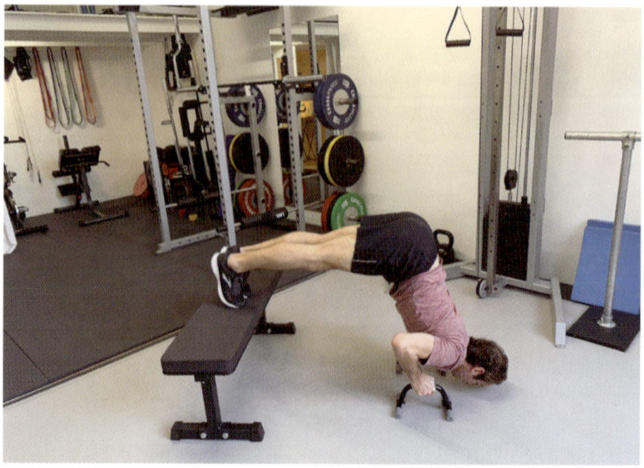

Fig. 147 Mid-movement.

UPPER-BODY EXERCISES

1. Start by finding the correct distance from the wall which is roughly a hand to a hand-and-a-half measurement away from the wall (Fig. 148).
2. Kick up into the handstand.
3. Keeping your legs together and core braced (Fig. 149), begin the descent by bending at the elbows until your head touches the ground, then push yourself back up (Fig. 150).
4. Be careful not to break form by collapsing through the back.
5. You can increase the difficulty of this by increasing the ROM with parallettes.

Dips

Dips are a fantastic upper body exercise and there are many variations of them. They work mainly the triceps and pectorals; however, the shoulders and core must work to stabilize the body during the movement.

1. Begin by getting into your starting position.
2. Your hands should be close to your sides – not too far away as this increases strain on the pectorals and shoulder girdle in the bottom position.
3. Depending on how much space there is below you, you can either have your legs in front or behind (Fig. 151).

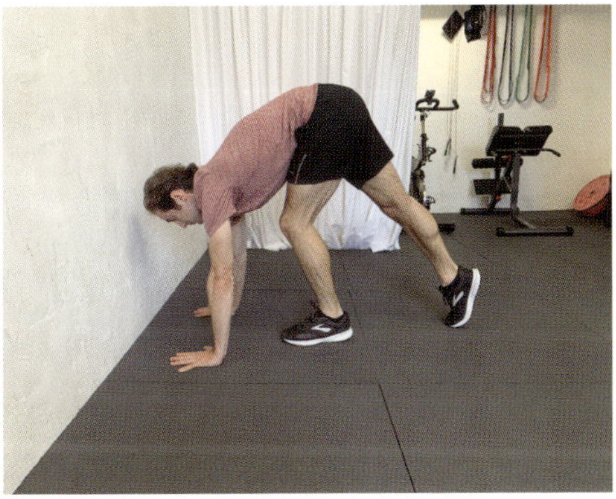

Fig. 148 Handstand set-up position.

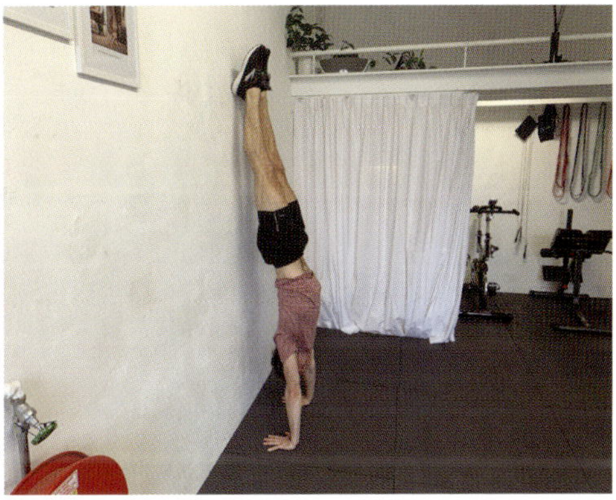

Fig. 149 Start position.

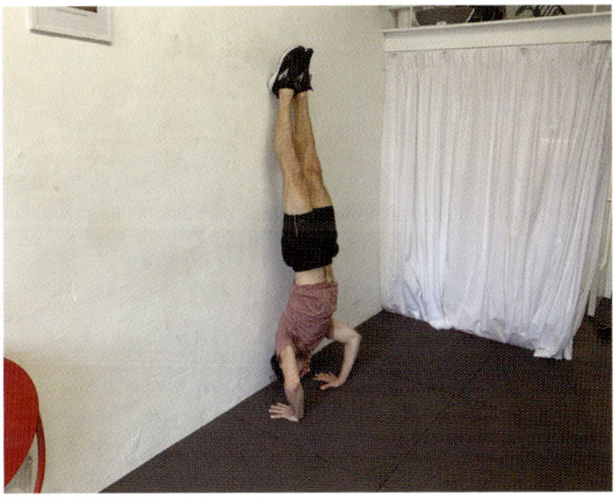

Fig. 150 Mid-movement.

125

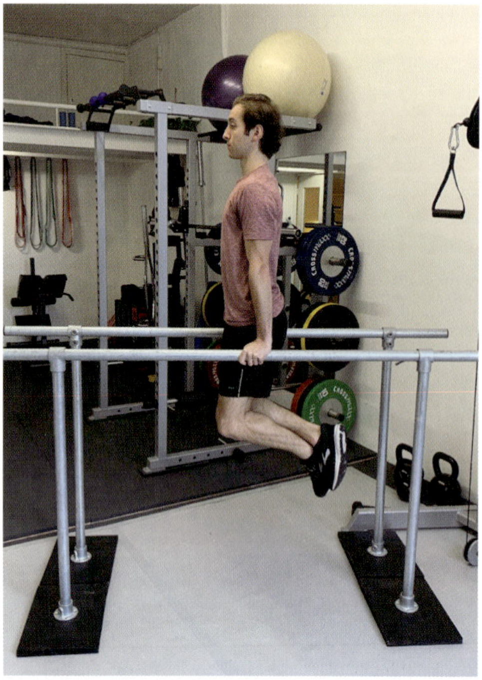

UPPER-BODY EXERCISES

Fig. 151 Dips start position.

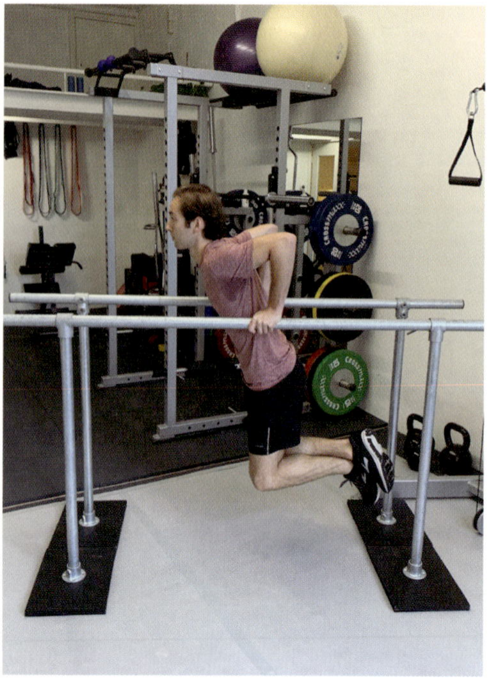

Fig. 152 Mid-movement.

4. Begin the descent by bending your elbows towards the back (not the side), and go as deep as your range allows.
5. In the bottom position your forearms and biceps should touch (Fig. 152).
6. Once there, begin to push yourself away from the bars and into your beginning lock-out position.
7. Repeat for the required number of repetitions.

Assisted chin-ups

This is a great way to introduce chin-ups as it allows a very graded approach and can be made progressively harder in small increments. You can do this a number of ways, here we have used the example shown.

1. Start by setting the pins at the desired height and placing a band around the pins (there are different strengths of bands so find one that's right for you).
2. If the squat rack you are using is high, place a bench next to it so that you can reach the bar and place yourself comfortably before you begin (Fig. 153).
3. Place your hands on the bars and feet in the band (Fig. 154).
4. Start the movement by pulling the shoulders down, then pull the elbows down, as far as your anatomy allows, squeezing the shoulder blades together; your chest should touch the bar at the top and you should be squeezing your mid-back hard with your elbows by your midline (Fig. 155).
5. Release your elbows from the position and let them extend.
6. As you come to end range, let the shoulders rise until you are at the starting position.
7. Keep a light brace throughout the exercise.
8. Repeat for the required number of repetitions.

UPPER-BODY EXERCISES

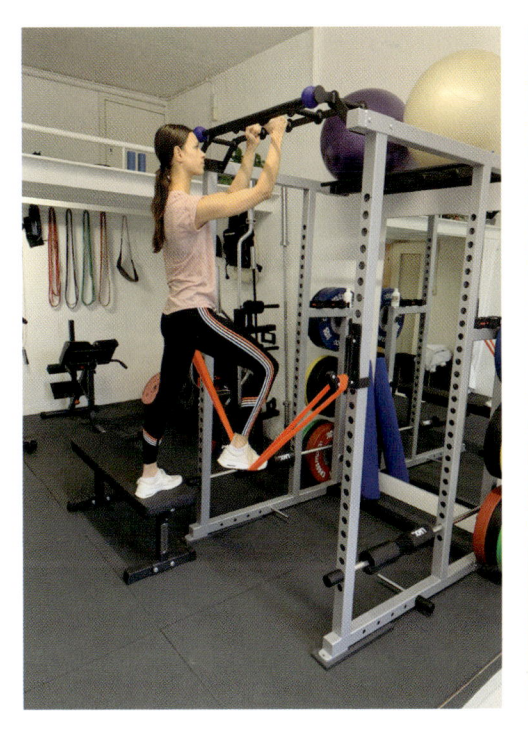

Fig. 153 Assisted chin-up set-up position.

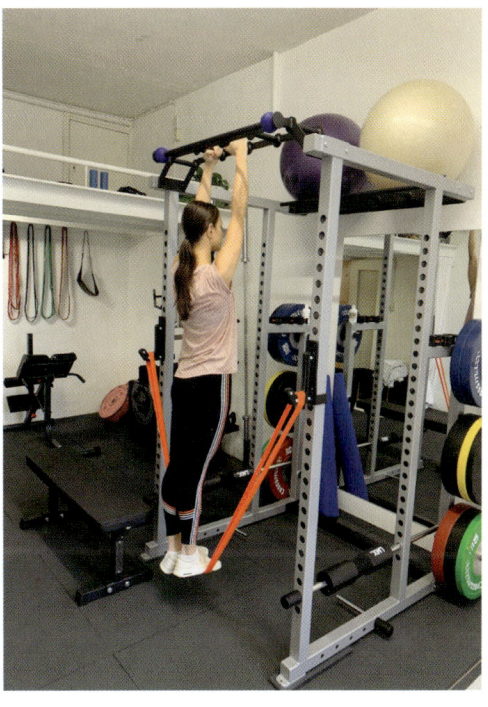

Fig. 154 Start position.

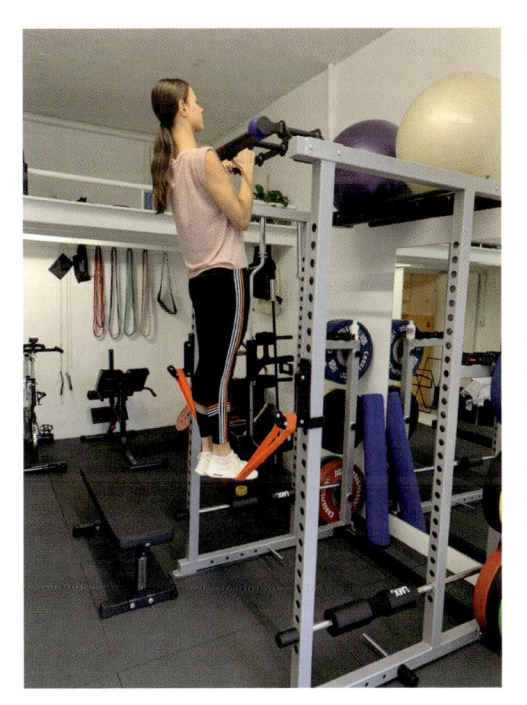

Fig. 155 Mid-movement.

Chin-ups

The difference between a chin-up and a pull-up is hand position. Chin-ups can have a neutral grip (palms facing each other), or a supinated grip (palms facing you). Pull-ups have the hands in a pronated grip (palms facing away from you). The primary focus of these exercises is on the latissimus dorsi and musculature of the mid-back.

We will use a neutral grip (palms facing each other), for this demonstration, as for most it is the strongest position to be in, as you will use much more of your biceps and forearms in comparison to other versions of this exercise. It is a great way to build upper back strength and can be performed almost anywhere there is a bar to hang from.

1. Place your hands on the bar with your palms facing each other and put your feet slightly in front (Fig. 156). This will activate your core a little and reduce sway when performing the exercise.

UPPER-BODY EXERCISES

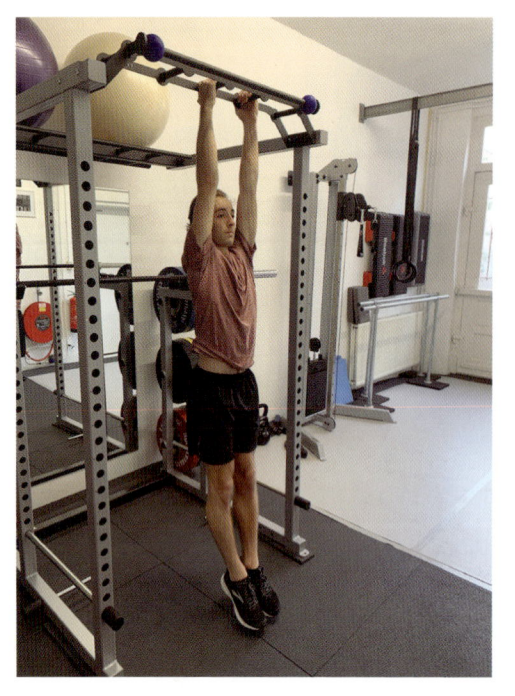

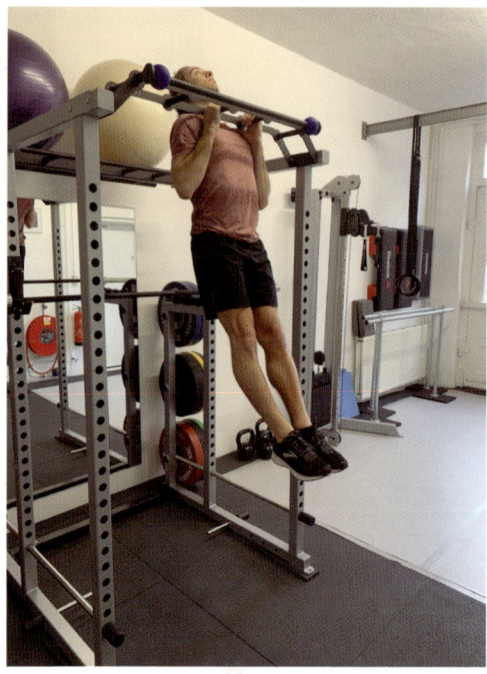

Fig. 156 Chin-up start position.

Fig. 157 Mid-movement.

2. Start the movement by pulling the shoulders down, then pull the elbows down as well, as far as your anatomy allows squeezing the shoulder blades together, your chest should touch the bar at the top and you should be squeezing your mid-back hard with your elbows by your midline (Fig. 157).
3. Release your elbows from the position and let them extend.
4. As you come to end range let the shoulders rise until you are at the starting position.
5. Repeat for the required number of repetitions.

Pull-ups

Place your hands on the bar just outside shoulder width with your palms facing away from you and put your feet slightly in front (Fig. 158), this will activate your core a little and reduce sway when performing the exercise.

1. Start the movement by pulling the shoulders down, then pull yourself towards the bar by bending at the elbow until you have reached your end range of motion, squeezing the shoulder blades together.
2. Your chin should clear the bar and ideally you want your chest to touch it at the top (Fig. 159).
3. Slowly begin to descend by extending your elbows from their position and as you come to end range let the shoulders rise until you are in your starting position.
4. Repeat for the required number of repetitions.

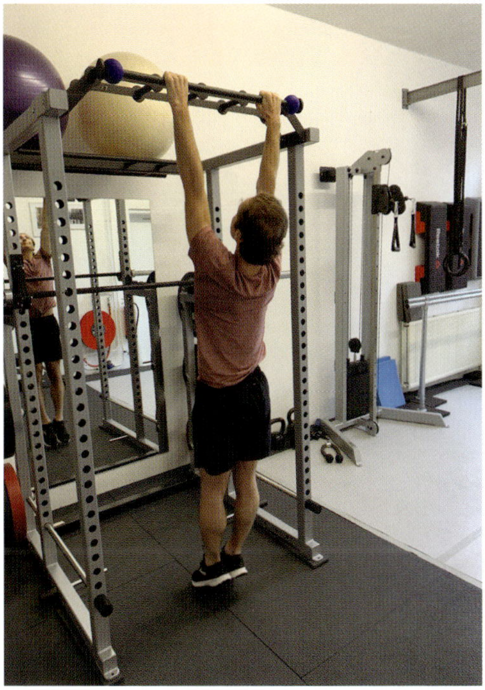

UPPER-BODY EXERCISES

Fig. 158 Pull-up start position.

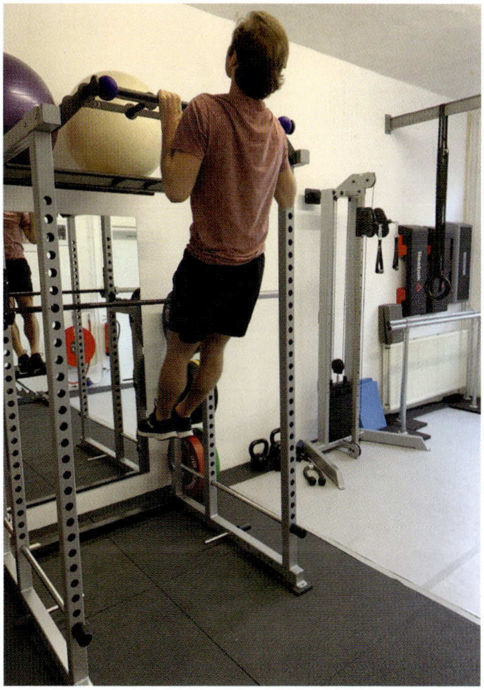

Fig. 159 Mid-movement.

RESISTANCE EQUIPMENT

Flat dumbbell press

The dumbbell press trains mainly the pectoralis major and triceps. By changing the position of the elbows, you can change the focus on whether you want more triceps or pectoralis major.

1. Take a pair of dumbbells and sit at the edge of a bench (Fig. 160).
2. As you lie back, bring the dumbbells up towards your shoulders.
3. When in your starting position (Fig. 161), take a breath, drive your feet into the ground, squeeze your glutes and lightly brace your core.
4. Push the dumbbells away from you while keeping your mid-back against the bench.
5. Do not overarch your low back and be careful not to let your hips come off it (Fig. 162).
6. Slowly lower the dumbbells towards your shoulders until they reach the beginning position.
7. Repeat for the required number of repetitions.

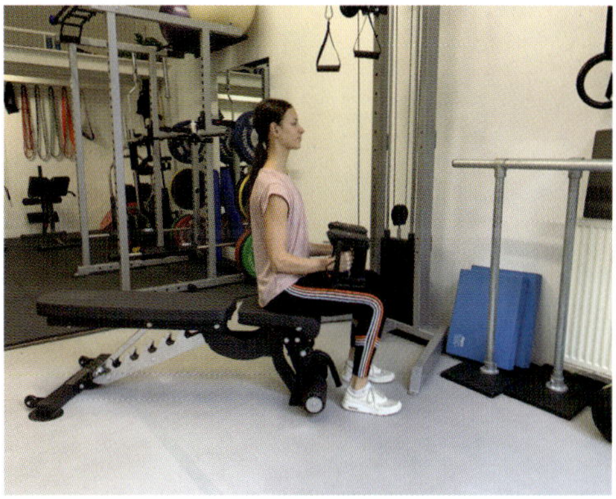

Fig. 160 Flat dumbbell press set-up position.

UPPER-BODY EXERCISES

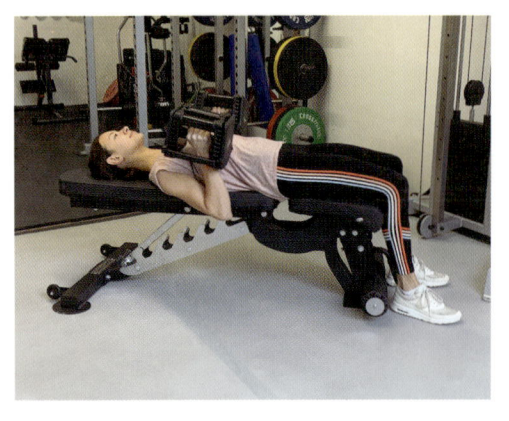

Fig. 161 Start position.

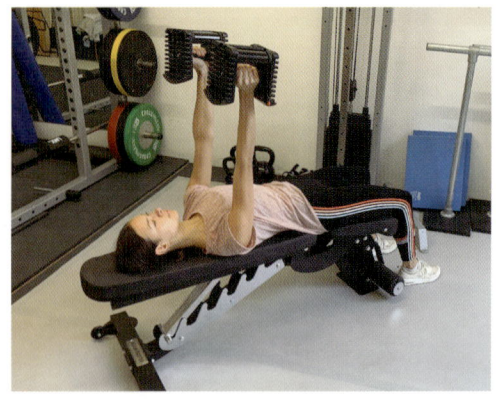

Fig. 162 Mid-movement.

Incline dumbbell press

Much the same as a flat dumbbell press; however, depending on the degree the focus shifts more toward the pectoralis minor and shoulders.

1. Set the bench at the angle you want.
2. Take a pair of dumbbells and sit at the edge of a bench (Fig. 163).
3. As you lie back bring the dumbbells up towards your shoulders (Fig. 164).
4. When in your starting position, take a breath, drive your feet into the ground, squeeze your glutes, lightly brace your core and push the dumbbells away from you (Fig. 165).
5. Slowly lower the dumbbells towards your shoulders until they reach the beginning position.
6. Repeat for the required number of repetitions.

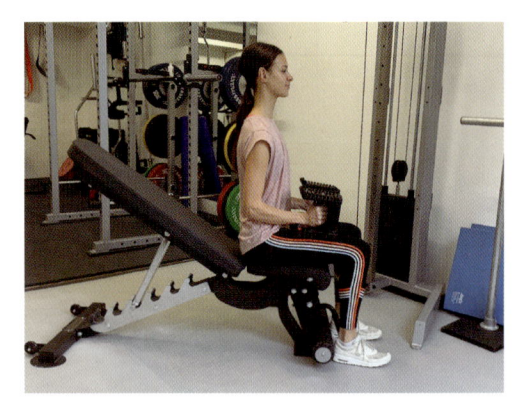

Fig. 163 Incline dumbbell press set-up position.

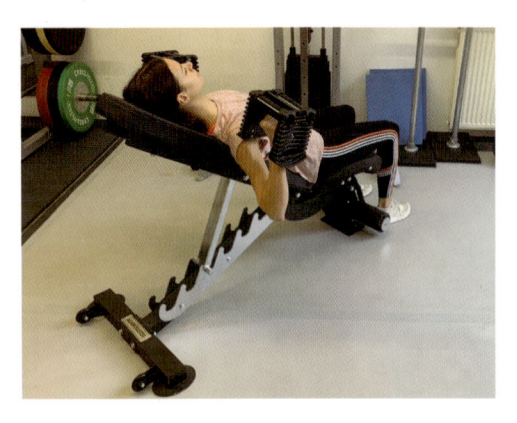

Fig. 164 Start position.

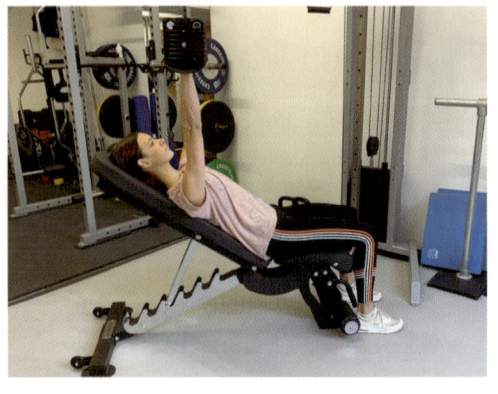

Fig. 165 Mid-movement.

130

UPPER-BODY EXERCISES

Seated overhead press

This exercise focuses on the shoulders and can be done with or without the support of a bench behind you. With the bench you will be able to load it more as it takes away the stability component required by the core. You can also do this as a single arm exercise.

1. Select the appropriate weight and sit with your legs either side of the bench.
2. Lift the dumbbells so they are resting on your shoulder with your elbows flared out to the side (Fig. 166).
3. Take a breath and brace your core then push the dumbbells up above your head until you reach lockout (Fig. 167).
4. Return them to the starting position and repeat.

Standing overhead press

This is just one example of an overhead press exercise; there are numerous versions, such as using kettlebells or landmines instead of barbells and dumbbells, and these can be done in various ways using both arms, or the single-arm versions and with differing positions. The primary focus of the overhead press is the shoulders and triceps, although the serratus anterior and trunk play a role in stabilization.

1. Much like the set-up for a front squat, the bar should be set in the pins at just below shoulder level (Fig. 168). This allows the person performing the exercise to clear the pins when un-racking and re-racking the bar.
2. Once this has been done, stand in front of the bar, walk towards it and place the bar on top of the upper portion of your chest.
3. Place your hands on the bar just outside of shoulder width, here the elbows can be pointed out slightly and they are facing down (unlike in the front rack position of the front squat).

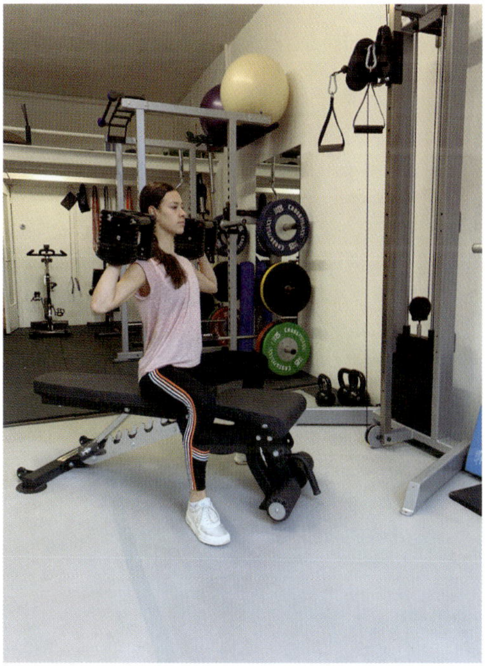

Fig. 166 Seated overhead press start position.

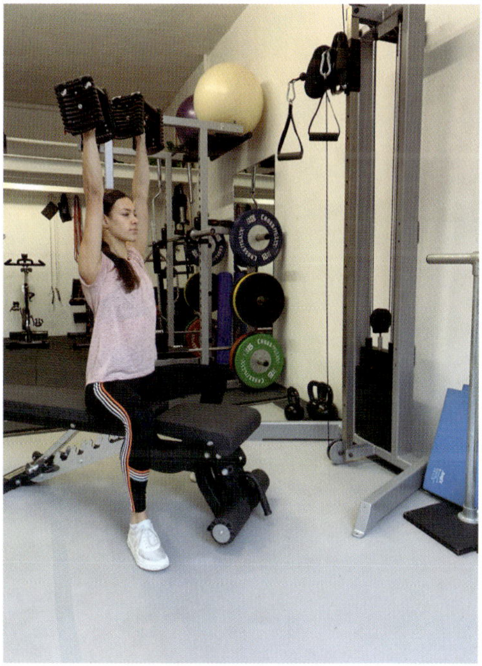

Fig. 167 Mid-movement.

UPPER-BODY EXERCISES

4. Take a step back out of the rack.
5. You can either use a split stance (Fig. 169), or bilateral one depending on what you prefer and what has been programmed.
6. Take a big breath and brace your core. As you go to raise the bar above your head you will have to lean back ever so slightly to clear your face.
7. Once you have done this, continue pushing the bar until you reach lockout and your arms are in line with your ears (Fig. 170).
8. The motion of the bar is somewhat akin to an upside down letter J.
9. As you begin to lower the bar you will again have to lean back a little to clear the bar from your face and then rest it on your chest.
10. Repeat for the number of repetitions.
11. Re-rack the bar.

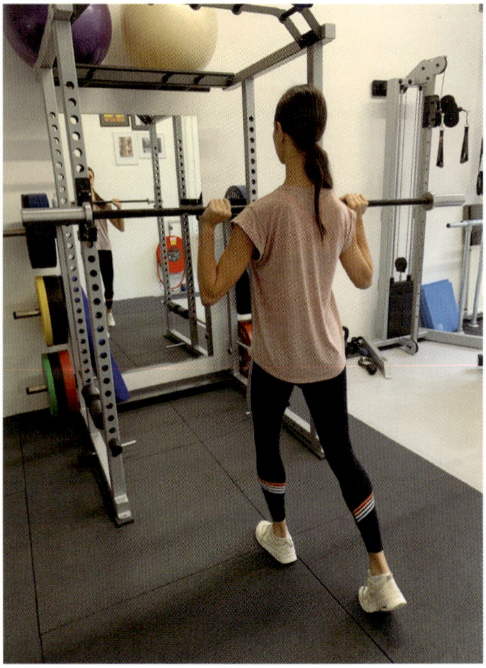

Fig. 169 Start position.

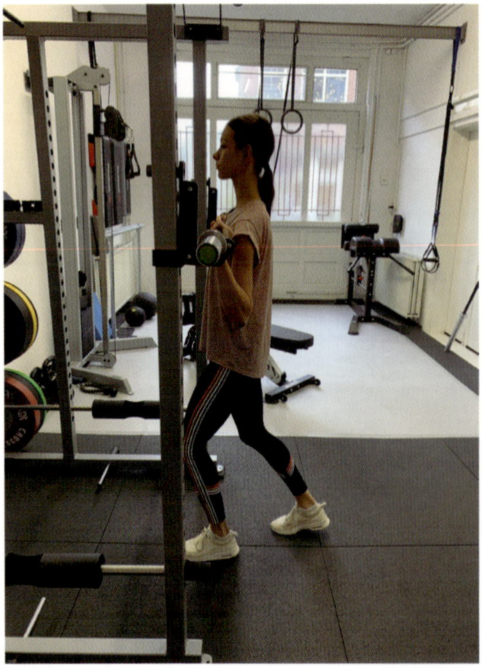

Fig. 168 Standing overhead press set-up position.

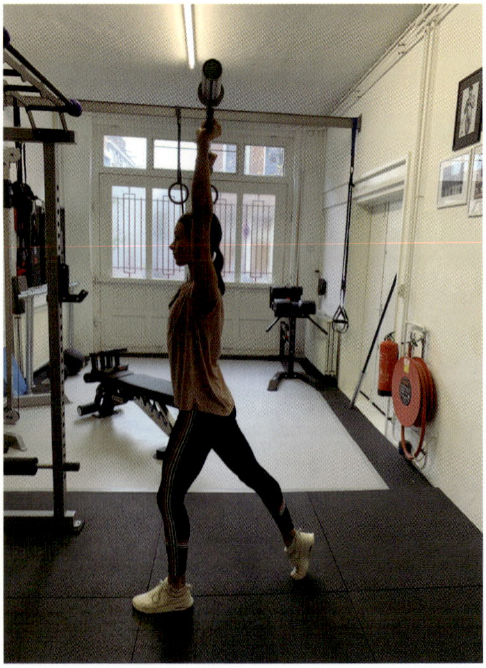

Fig. 170 Mid-movement.

UPPER-BODY EXERCISES

Kneeling single arm cable row

This is a good place to start when it comes to training the mid-back, which consists of the rhomboids and mid-trapezius, as well as training the latissimus dorsi.

1. Place the cable at its highest point with the handle attachment and set the weight at the required amount.
2. Take the handle in the arm that you want to work and walk back until the weight stack has risen and there is tension on the cable.
3. Get into a half kneeling position with the arm extended in front of you (Fig. 171).
4. The movement should begin first at the shoulder blade with retraction and then the elbow should move backwards until you hit your end range without any shoulder elevation (Fig. 172).
5. Once there begin to straighten the arm all the while keeping the shoulder-blade in place until the very last moment when it should protract (go forward).
6. The easiest way to remember this is to think of the shoulder-blades as good students: they are the first in and the last out.

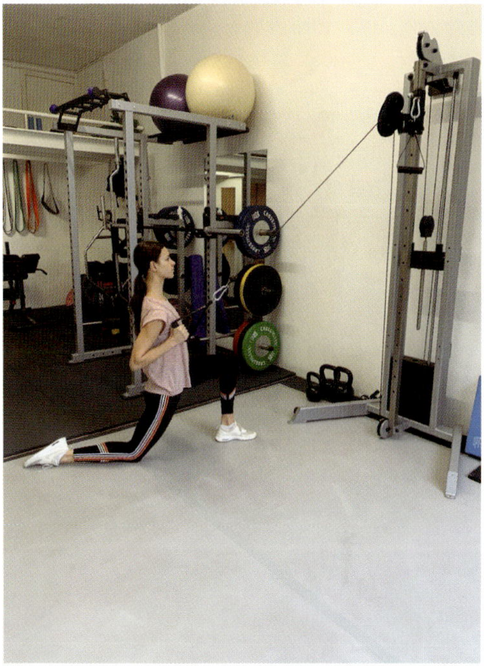

Fig. 172 Mid-movement.

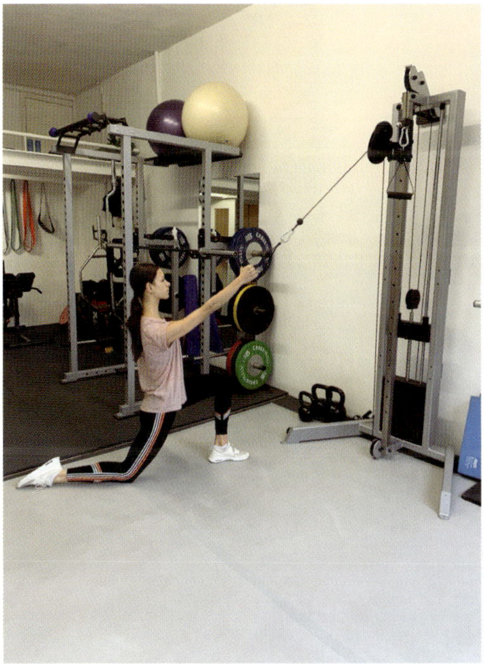

Fig. 171 Kneeling single arm cable row start position.

Chest supported incline dumbbell row

This exercise trains the mid-back and lats. It can be very useful for those suffering from low back pain as it takes the load off of this area so that you can focus on the muscles being worked.

1. Put a bench at the angle that you want and lower yourself forward onto it, making sure that your head and neck are clear.
2. Take the dumbbells in each hand from the ground (Fig. 173).
3. Squeeze your glutes to keep them active throughout the movement.

133

UPPER-BODY EXERCISES

4. Initiate the movement by retracting the scapulae and then pull the elbows towards your midline as far as your anatomy allows, squeezing the shoulder blades together (Fig. 174).
5. Gently release your elbows from the position and let them extend. As you come to end range, let the scapulae move forward until you are at the starting position.
6. Make sure that you keep your core braced throughout the exercise.
7. Repeat for the required number of repetitions.

Single arm dumbbell row

This exercise is a great mid-back strengthener and also acts somewhat as an anti-rotational exercise for the core. It can be used with different hand, elbow and torso positions to create differing stimulus to the muscles worked.

1. Put one knee and one hand on a bench.
2. The knee should be in line with your hips and your wrist in line with your shoulder.
3. Your stance leg should be just wide enough to create a good base, so that your hips are equal in height and your back is in a good neutral position.
4. Take the dumbbell from the ground in the arm that will be worked (Fig. 175).
5. Initiate the movement by retracting the scapula and then pull the elbow towards your midline as far as your anatomy allows (Fig. 176).
6. Gently release your elbow from the position and let it extend.
7. As you come to end range let the scapula move forwards until you are at the starting position.
8. Make sure to keep your core braced throughout the exercise.
9. Repeat for the required number of repetitions.

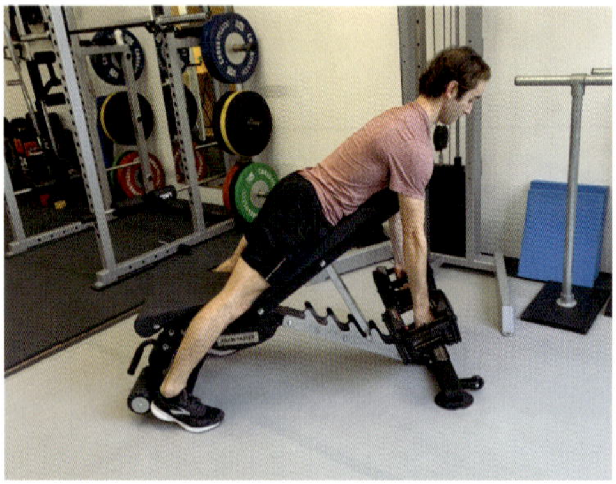

Fig. 173 Chest supported incline dumbbell row start position.

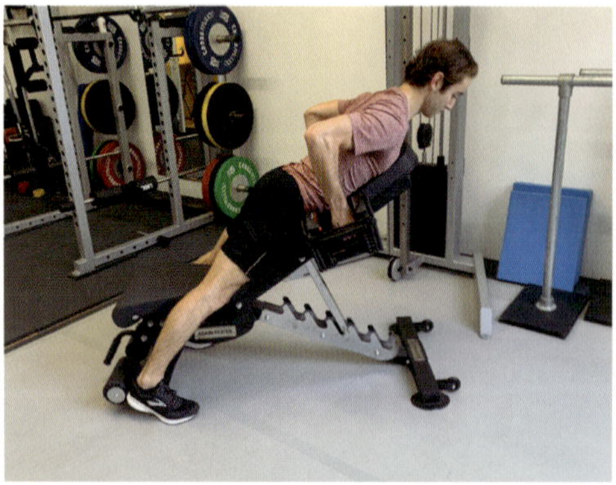

Fig. 174 Mid-movement.

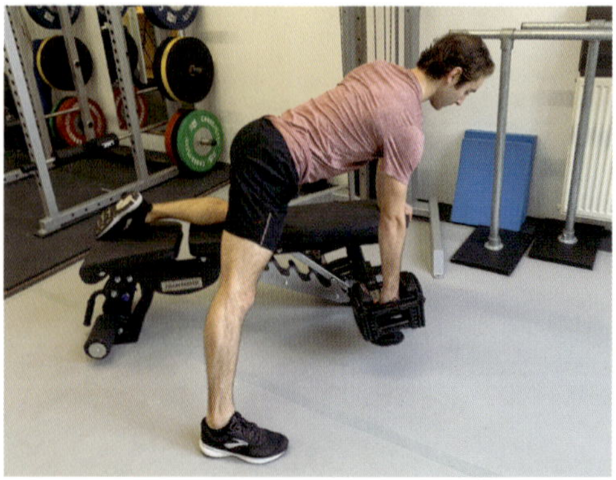

Fig. 175 Single arm dumbbell row start position.

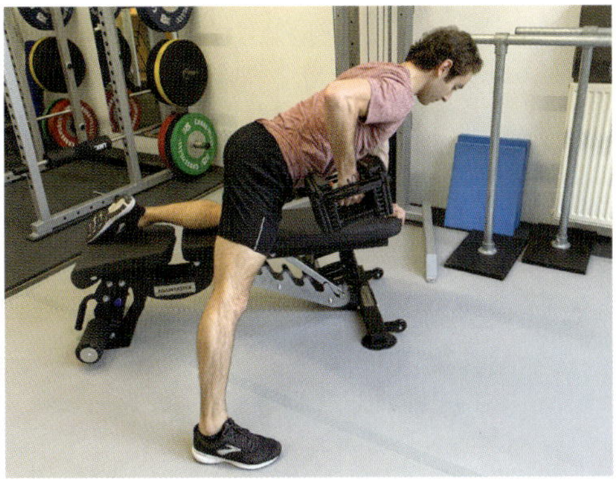

UPPER-BODY EXERCISES

Fig. 176 Mid-movement.

Bilateral seated row

This exercise trains the latissimus dorsi, rhomboids and trapezius muscles. It also has an indirect training effect on the erectors as they must stay upright in order to maintain good form.

Depending on the machine you have at your disposal you may be able to place your feet in front of you on the supports. If this is the case, place them low as this allows a little more freedom in the hips (in this version we are placing the feet behind the bench supports as the bench is heavy enough, to make sure we create a good amount of resistance to pull from).

1. Take the bar in both hands and get into position (Fig. 177).
2. Keep a gentle brace throughout the exercise.
3. Initiate the movement by retracting the scapulae and then pull the elbows backwards as far as your anatomy allows squeezing the shoulder blades tightly together, making sure that there is no shoulder elevation (Fig. 178).
4. Release your elbows from the position and let them extend. As you come to end range, let the scapulae move forward until you are at the starting position.
5. Be careful not to sway back and forth using your torso to create momentum during this exercise, as this takes focus away from the muscles that it is directed towards.
6. Repeat for the required number of repetitions.

Bilateral bent-over row

The bent-over row can be done in a number of different ways with a number of different devices. Here we will use the barbell version. It is a good way to train the mid-back in a nice dynamic way while engaging the posterior chain in an isometric fashion.

If you have a squat rack with pins, set them at the height of your extended position for the row.

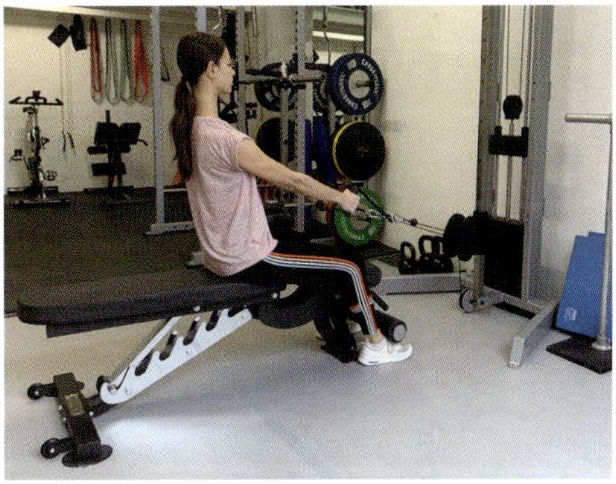

Fig. 177 Bilateral seated row start position.

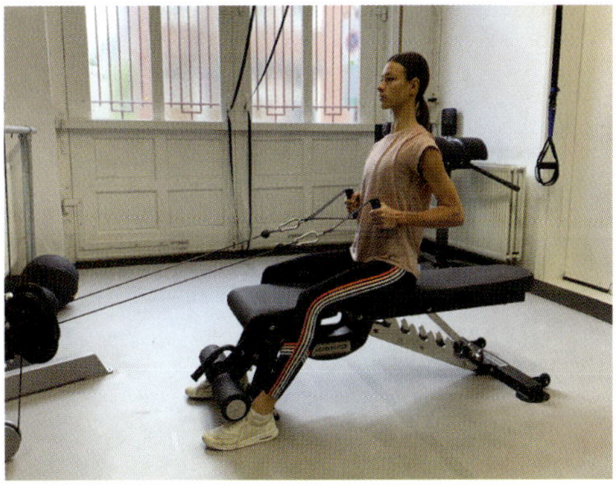

Fig. 178 Mid-movement.

UPPER-BODY EXERCISES

1. Stand in front of the barbell and get into a good hip hinge position of between roughly 70 and 90 degrees. If you are any higher, you risk the exercise becoming more of a shrug, which is more for the upper trapezius, than a row.
2. Take an overhand grip (you can also perform this with a supinated grip), with your hands just outside of shoulder width (Fig. 179).
3. Lift the weight off the pins and begin.
4. As with any row, begin the movement from the shoulder blades and then the elbows.
5. Make sure to squeeze the shoulder blades together in the most concentric part of the movement (Fig. 180), before returning to your starting position.

Single arm lat pulldown

This exercise focuses on the latissimus dorsi, although it does also train the muscles of the mid-back. It can be used a number of ways, which makes it an extremely versatile exercise.

1. Set yourself up so that you are seated in a nice straight position with your arm overhead and fully extended and the shoulder elevated (Fig. 181).
2. As with any pulling movement, begin by pulling the shoulder down first then bend at the elbow until you have reached end range (Fig. 182).
3. Return to your starting position.
4. Repeat for the required number of repetitions.

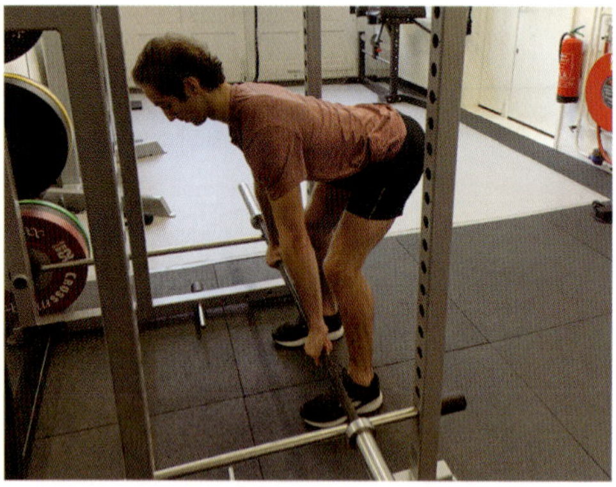

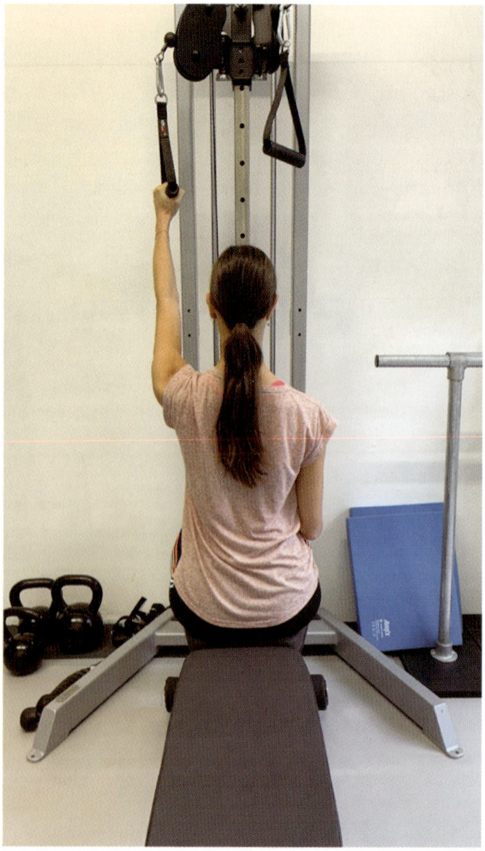

Fig. 179 Bilateral bent-over row start position.

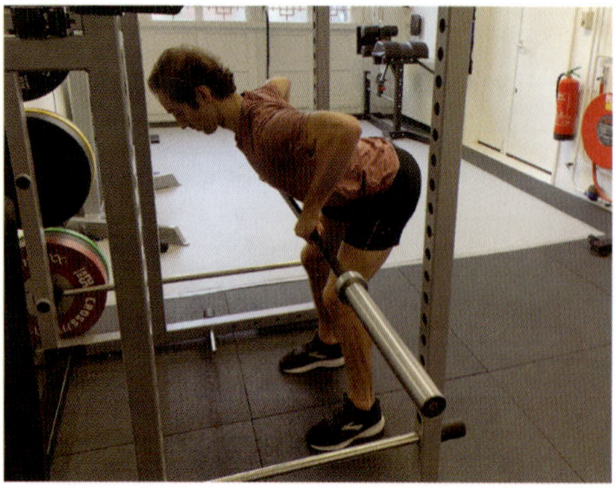

Fig. 180 Mid-movement.

Fig. 181 Single arm lat pulldown start position.

UPPER-BODY EXERCISES

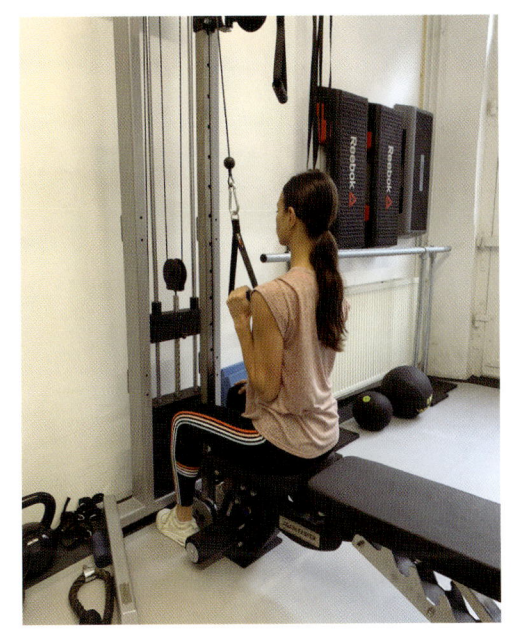

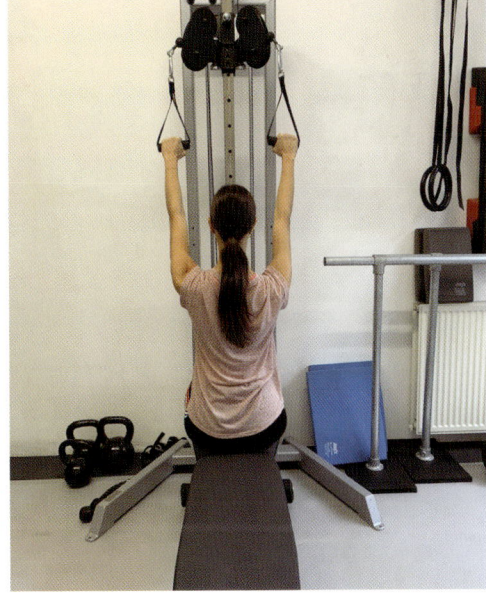

Fig. 182 Mid-movement.

Fig. 183 Bilateral lat pulldown start position.

Bilateral lat pulldowns

You can perform this exercise in a number of different ways using different hand positions as well as different implements.

1. Set the pin at the selected weight.
2. Take the handles in your hands with your palms facing away from you outside of shoulder width (Fig. 183).
3. Lean back ever so slightly and start the movement by pulling the shoulders down, then pull the elbows down as well, as far as your anatomy allows, squeezing the shoulder blades together (Fig. 184).
4. Release your elbows from the position and let them extend.
5. As you come to end range, let the shoulders rise until you are at the starting position.
6. Be careful not to sway back and forth using your torso to create momentum during this exercise as this takes focus away from the muscles that it is directed towards.
7. Keep a light brace throughout the exercise.
8. Repeat for the required number of repetitions.

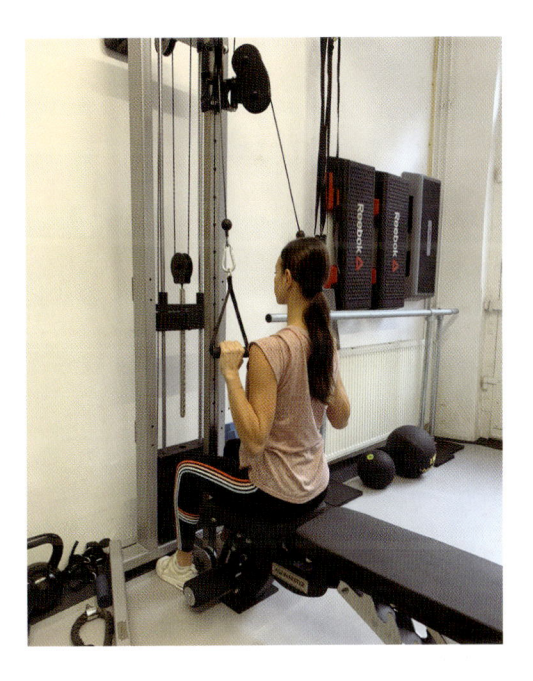

Fig. 184 Mid-movement.

9 PLYOMETRICS

As mentioned previously in this book, these exercises are high force and should not be done when tired. It is also really important to focus on minimizing the time between the muscle lengthening and muscle shortening phases (eccentric and concentric phases).

LOWER BODY PLYOMETRICS

Jump rope/skipping

Jump rope or skipping is what is known as an 'extensive plyometric' meaning that it is sub-maximal in nature and a great way to introduce this type of training into a dancer's workload without burdening the system too much and at the same time adding volume. This exercise helps prepare the body, especially the ankle complex, for the higher-level demands of other plyometrics training.

Ideally you want as short a ground contact time as possible. Depending on the outcome you or your trainer want to achieve, there are a number of ways to perform this exercise; in this example, we are going for little to no heel contact with the ground and small jumps which can be performed for time or repetitions.

The first thing you'll want is a good rope, which can be purchased from many different outlets; there is a vast choice of makes and types.

1. First, without using the rope, try the small jumps. Make sure that they are light and springy; practise the wrist movement along with it.
2. To perform the exercise with the rope, keep your hands close to your sides and slightly in front of you as this allows the rope a better arch for you to jump over (Fig. 185).
3. The movement must come mainly from your wrists and not too much arm movement.
4. Start with the rope behind you on the ground and then using your arms swing it overhead and jump over it (Fig. 186).
5. It will take a little practice, but the benefits of this exercise are many.

*Note: women should be aware that they may feel a sensation of wanting to go to the bathroom when performing this. If this is this case, stop the exercise and get yourself evaluated by a healthcare professional as you may have a pelvic floor dysfunction, which should be addressed before recommencing this exercise.

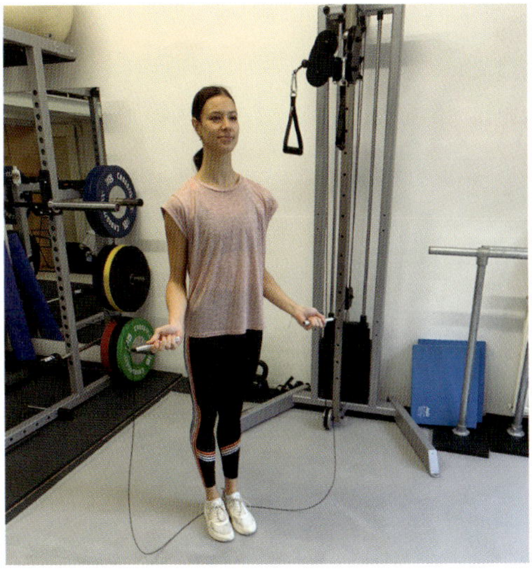

PLYOMETRICS

Fig. 185 Skipping start position.

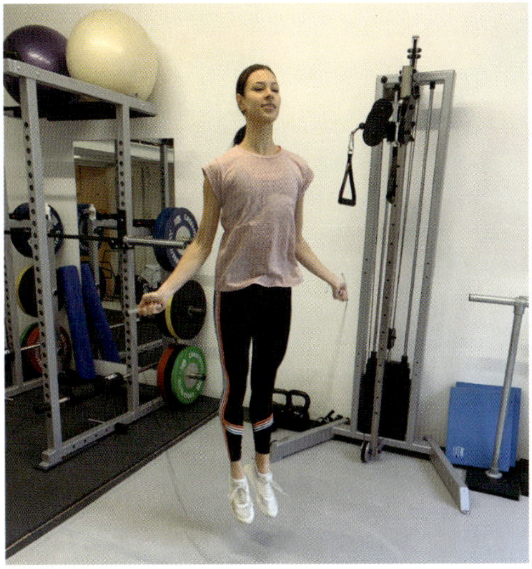

Fig. 186 Mid-movement.

Reverse drop jumps off a low step

This is an extensive short coupling plyometric. Due to the low step it serves to introduce differing impact levels to the body and continues to help strengthen the ankle complex. This exercise can be done for repetitions or time.

1. Start with a low step and jump on and off it repeatedly (Figs 187 and 188).
2. You can choose to use arms or not, depending on whether you want them involved.
3. After some training you can change the height; however, the idea is that you want as little ground contact time as possible with minimal to no heel contact.

Pogo-hops

Pogo-hops are a little more intense than jump rope. The idea behind it is to build momentum

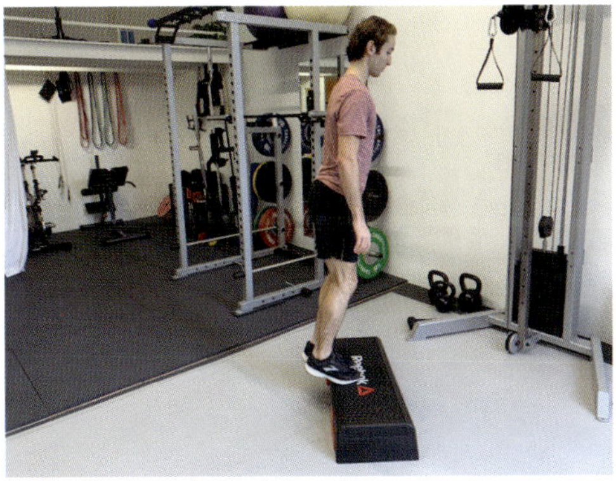

Fig. 187 Reverse drop jumps off a low step start position.

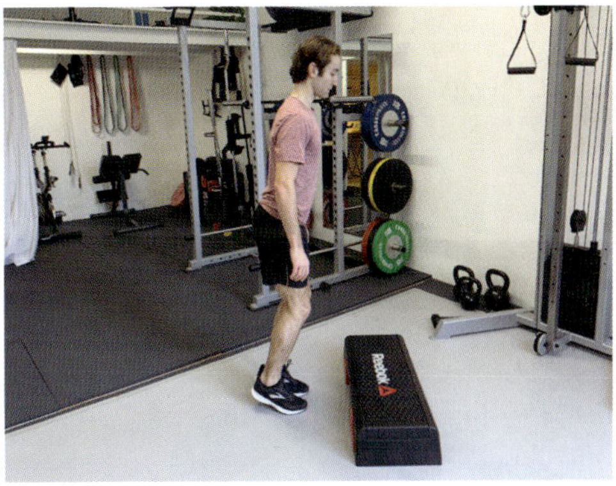

Fig. 188 Land position.

139

PLYOMETRICS

Fig. 189 Pogo-hops start position.

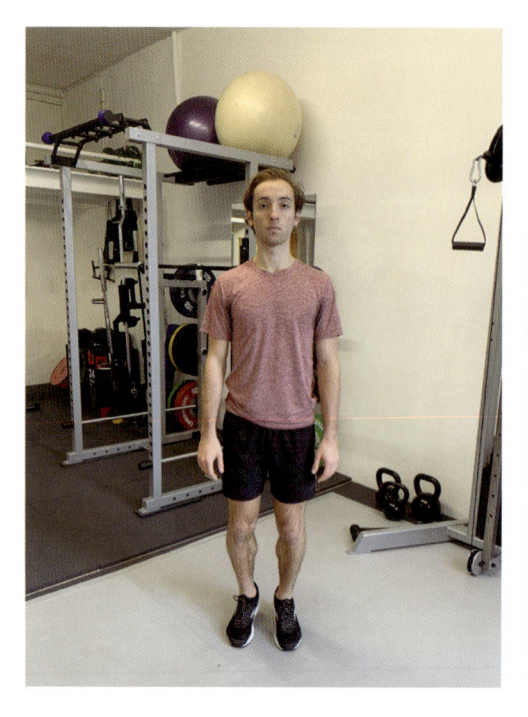

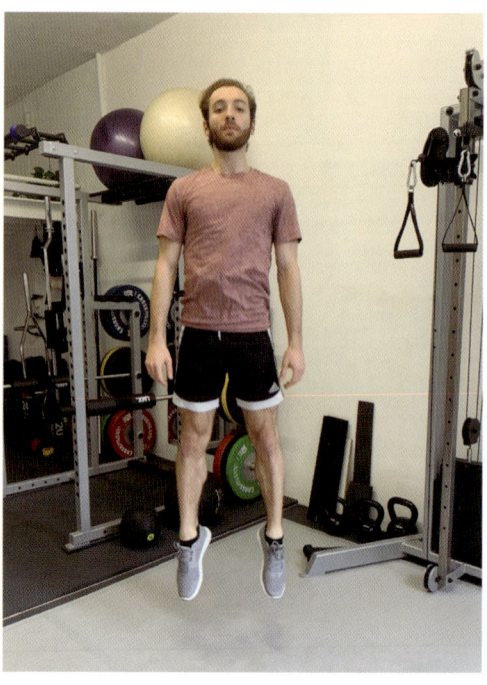

Fig. 190 Mid-movement.

so that your jump increases in height by using the elastic energy recoil that is being stored and released in the ankle complex.

1. Start nice and easy (Figs 189 and 190), and slowly build in intensity and jump height over a given number of repetitions and time.
2. You can use arm swing to help with the exercise.

Single leg push jumps on low step

This is a good exercise to begin with, as the impact on landing is lower due to the step whilst also teaching push off from the working leg.

1. Stand facing laterally with one foot on the step.
2. Raise the foot of the working leg (Fig. 191) and drop it down onto the step and push yourself up and away to explode up into the air, raising the knee of the opposite leg (Fig. 192).
3. Upon landing make sure to go through the whole foot from toes to heel and bend slightly at the knee and hip.
4. This can be done for repetitions or time.

Skater jumps (lateral movement)

Skater jumps are to help with lateral movement (which is extremely important in dance), as well as being more compliant* when it comes to jump training, as the knee and hip become much more involved.

(*Stiffness = minimal ground contact time; compliance = longer ground contact time.)

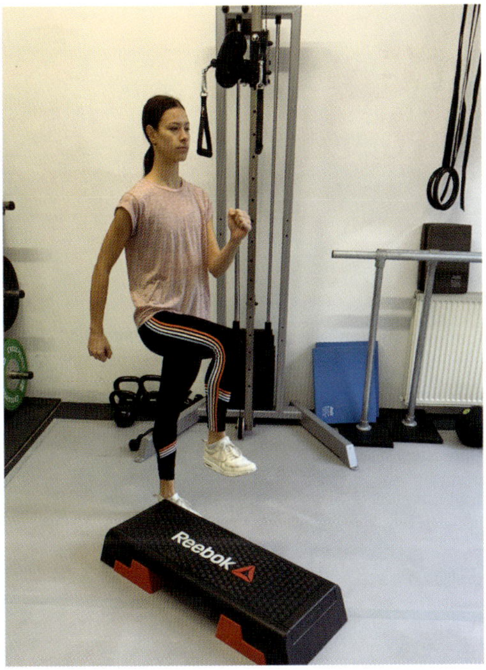

PLYOMETRICS

Fig. 191 Single leg push jumps on low step start position.

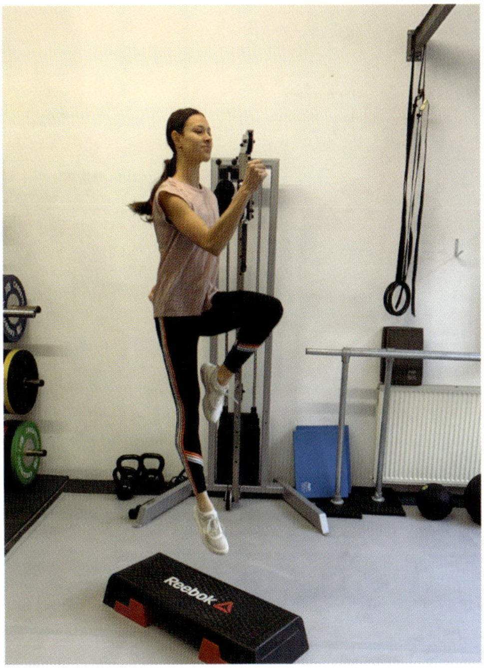

Fig. 192 Mid-movement.

1. Begin standing on one foot (Fig. 193) and jump sideways (Fig. 194) so that you land on the other foot.
2. As you land, make sure to keep the hips as square as possible, going through the whole foot and bending at the knee and hip (Fig. 195).
3. Push back through the foot to take off to jump to the other side.
4. This can be done for time or repetitions.

Box jumps

Box jumps are a great way to introduce much higher intensity plyometrics without the impact upon landing due to the box placement.

1. Set the box at the required height. Do not start too high, as the idea of these jumps is to jump as high as possible without your knees rising above your hips in the air and

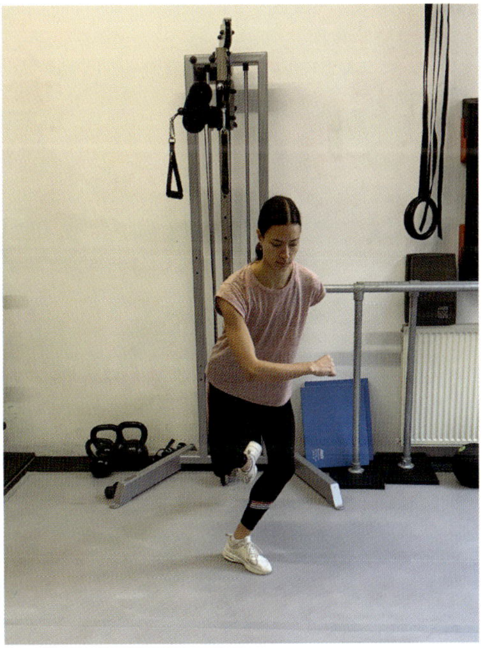

Fig. 193 Skater jump start position.

141

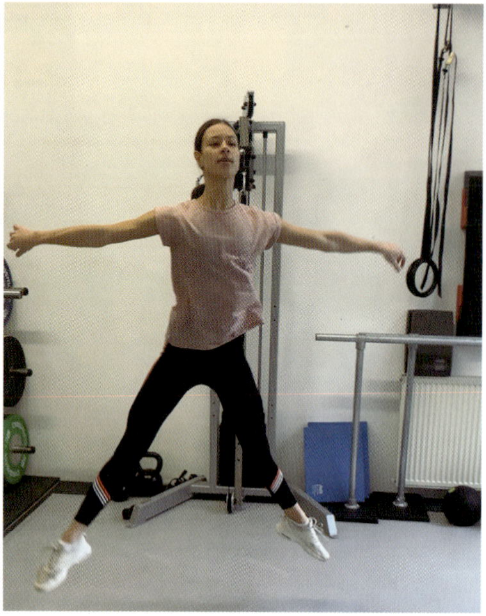

PLYOMETRICS

Fig. 194 Jump.

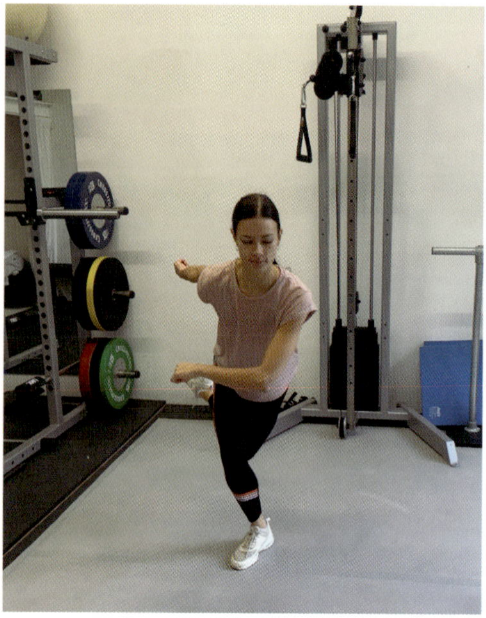

Fig. 195 Land position.

be able to land safely and effectively on the box.
2. Start in front of the box (Fig. 196).
3. Swing your arms back, bend at your hips and knees, then explode up (Fig. 197), and jump onto the box landing in a good, safe position, almost identical to the one that you took off from (Fig. 198).
4. Make sure to step down off the box and not jump down.
5. Repeat for the required number of repetitions.

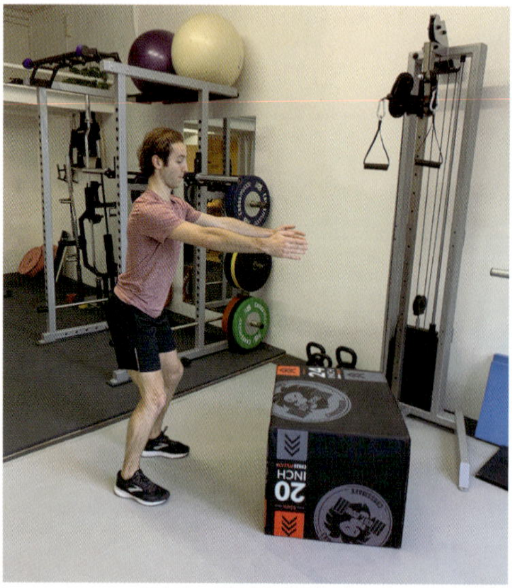

Fig. 196 Box jump start position.

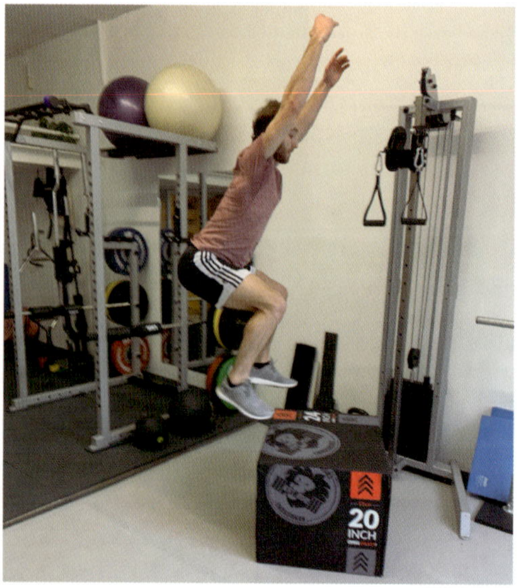

Fig. 197 Jump.

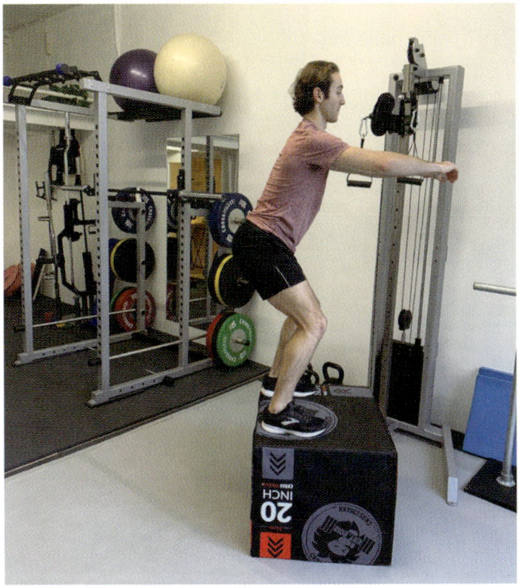

PLYOMETRICS

Fig. 198 Land position.

Squat jumps

These are great to teach starting and landing positions on the ground. These can be done with repeated efforts or by taking out the counter movement; in doing this you remove the elastic component. This depends entirely on the goal that you require.

1. Bring the arms back and behind you, bend at the knee and hip into a squat position (Fig. 199).
2. Explode up into the air and jump as high as you can (Fig. 200).
3. Upon landing return to your beginning squat position.

Depth jumps – rebounds

The idea behind these is to drop off a box, and upon landing, to use the elastic recoil as fast as possible to take off again, with minimal ground contact time (more stiffness), and minimal knee flexion and jump onto another box.

1. Place one foot out in front of you over the edge of the step (Fig. 201).

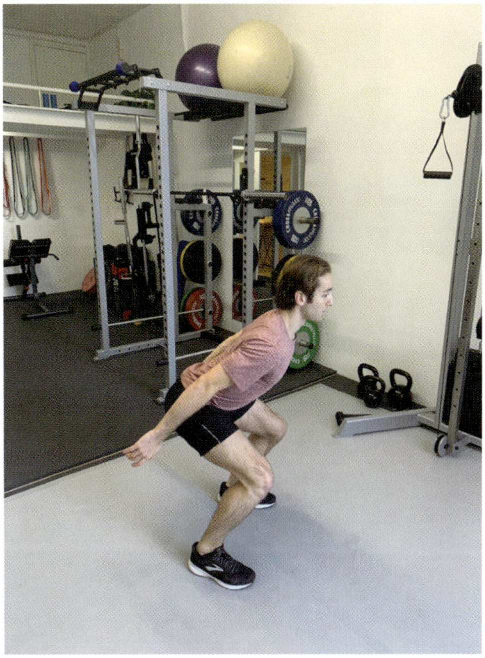

Fig. 199 Single leg push jumps on low step start position.

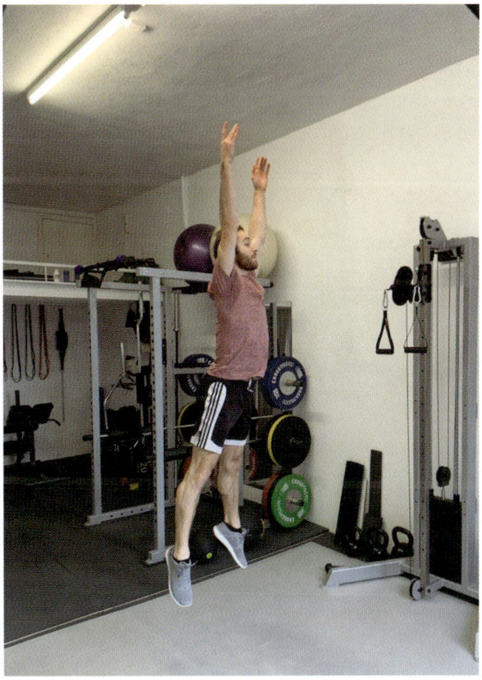

Fig. 200 Mid-movement.

143

PLYOMETRICS

2. Drop (don't jump) off the box.
3. As soon as your foot makes contact with the ground (Fig. 202), jump up towards the other box (Fig. 203), and then land (Fig. 204).
4. When repeating, walk back around to your starting box; this ensures that you have a small rest in between repetitions.

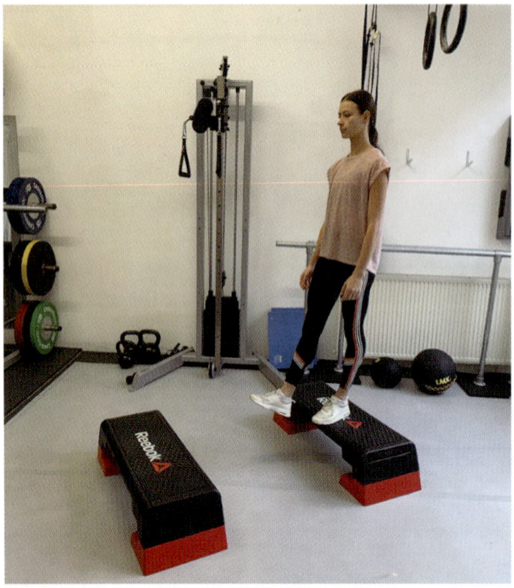

Fig. 201 Depth jump start position.

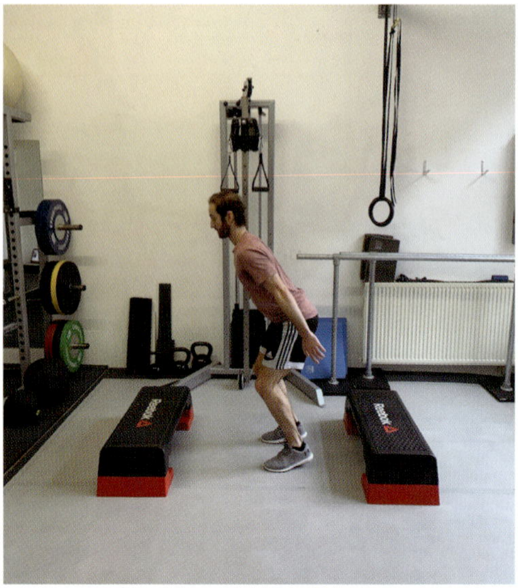

Fig. 202 Floor landing.

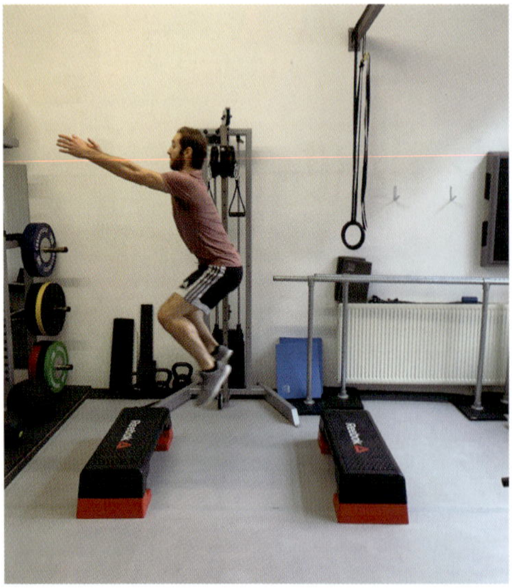

Fig. 203 Jump.

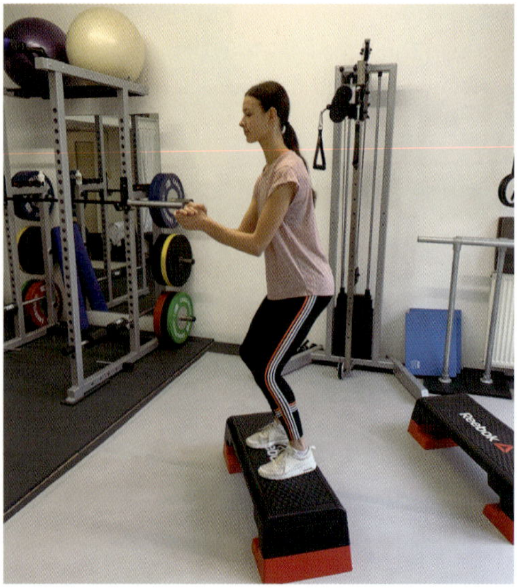

Fig. 204 Land position on box.

PLYOMETRICS

Depth jump

The difference between these two depth jumps is in the landing off the box.

1. Start by placing one foot out over the edge of the box with your arms in front of you (Fig. 205).
2. Drop, don't jump off the box.
3. When landing, land through the whole foot, bending at the knees and hips also this makes it more compliant.
4. Explode up as high as possible (Fig. 206), reaching triple extension (this means that the ankles, knees and hips are all in extension).
5. Once you've landed, step back on the box and repeat for the required number of repetitions.

UPPER BODY PLYOMETRICS

Plyometric push-ups

Plyometric push-ups are great to help with explosive strength in the upper body. You want to perform them as explosively as possible, until just before your speed and height begin to drop off.

1. Begin in a push-up position (Fig. 207).
2. Lower yourself quickly toward the ground and push up as fast as possible, letting your hands leave the ground (Fig. 208).
3. On the return drop down into the bottom position and explode up again.
4. Repeat until performance begins to slow. As soon as this happens the set is over, as the

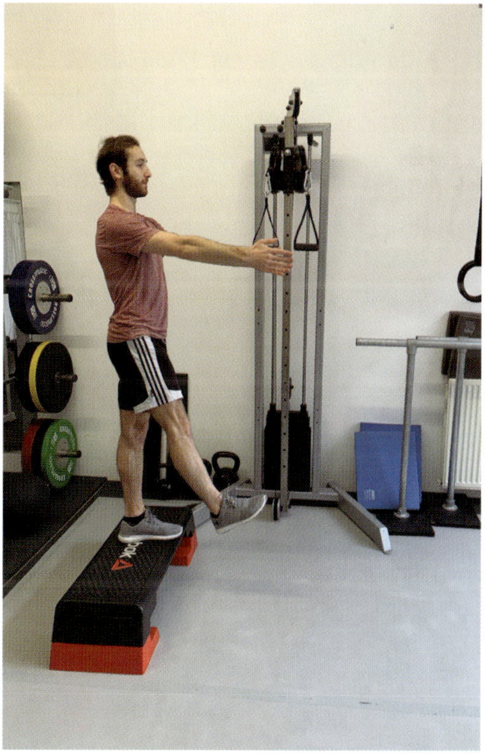

Fig. 205 Single leg push jumps on low step start position.

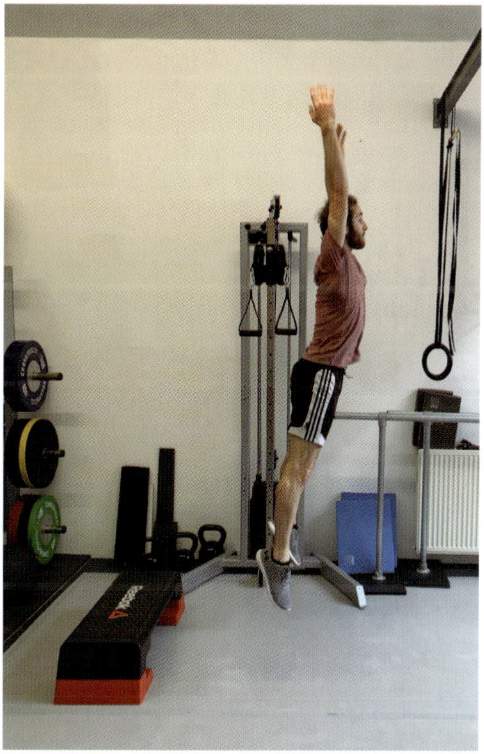

Fig. 206 Mid-movement.

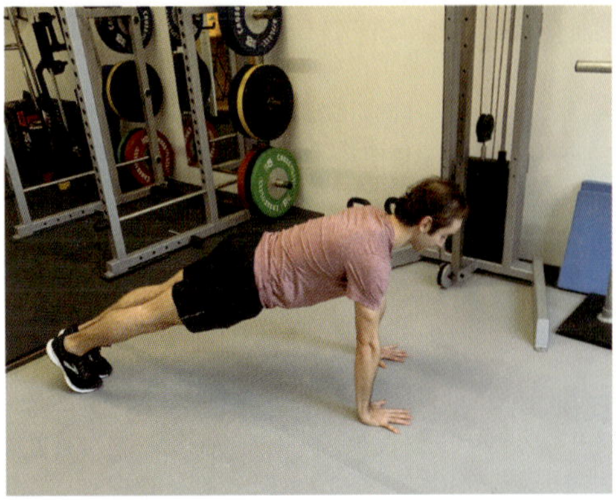

PLYOMETRICS

Fig. 207 Plyometric push-up start position.

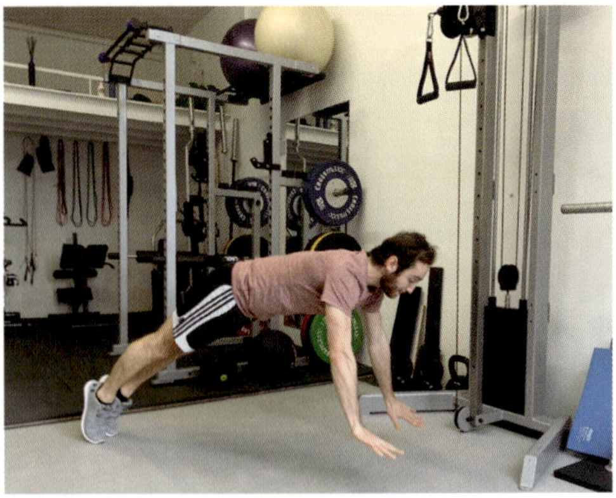

Fig. 208 Mid-movement.

idea of the exercise is to produce maximal force over the whole set.

Medicine ball throw

1. Stand facing a wall holding the medicine ball at chest height and far enough away so that when you throw the ball you can also catch and release it straight away (Fig. 209).

2. Press the ball away from you so that it hits the wall and bounces back towards you (Fig. 210).
3. Upon catching it, press it away again as fast as possible.
4. You can do this for time or repetitions.

This is the extensive version; it can also be done intensively, the difference being that you will stand further away from the wall and throw it as hard as you can against the wall and let it drop on the ground before picking it up and repeating it.

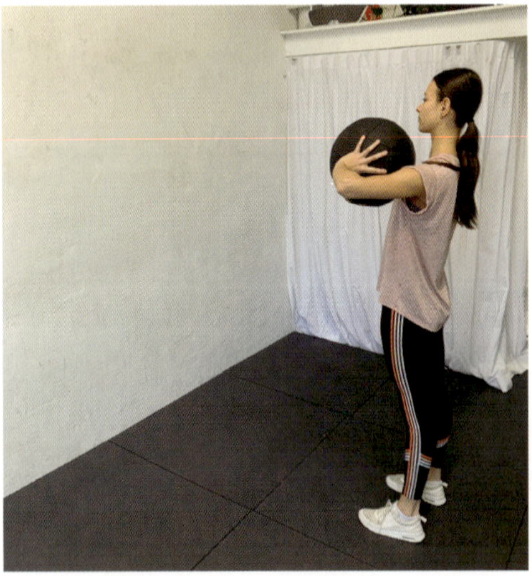

Fig. 209 Medicine ball throw start position.

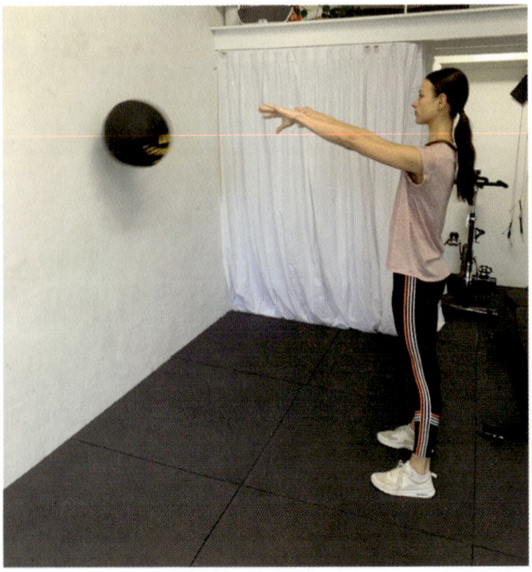

Fig. 210 End position.

Medicine ball oblique toss

Much like the sagittal plane medicine ball throw, this version can be done extensively or intensively. Here we will demonstrate the extensive version. The focus on this is the obliques.

1. Holding the ball in an underhand toss position (Fig. 211), stand sideways to the wall, holding close enough so that you can catch the ball once you've thrown it.
2. Throw the ball toward the wall (Fig. 212), and then catch and release it as quickly as possible in a rhythmic fashion.
3. This can be done for time or repetitions.

Medicine ball slams

This exercise is a great way to help production of upper body power.

1. Take a medicine ball and hold it overhead (Fig. 213).
2. Bring the ball down, throwing it at the ground as hard as you can.
3. Your knees and hips should be involved in this movement when performing it (Fig. 214).
4. Be careful to throw the ball slightly away from you so as not to have it come up and hit you.
5. Take the ball and repeat.
6. This can be performed for time or repetitions.

Medicine ball lateral slams

1. Take a medicine ball and hold it overhead (Fig. 215).
2. Bring the ball down and to one side, throwing it at the ground as hard as you can.

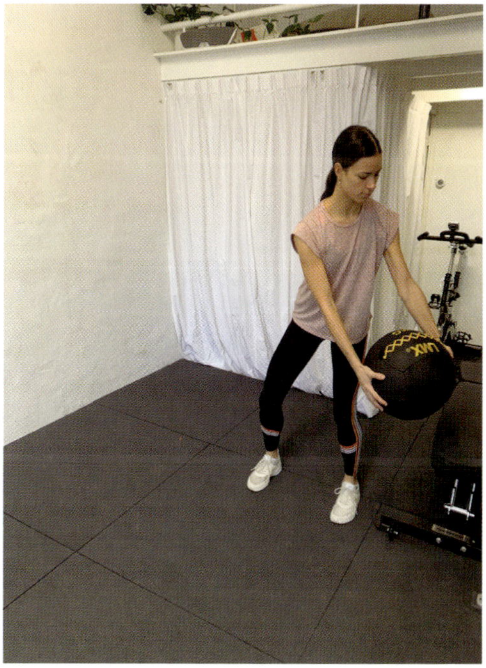

Fig. 211 Medicine ball oblique toss start position.

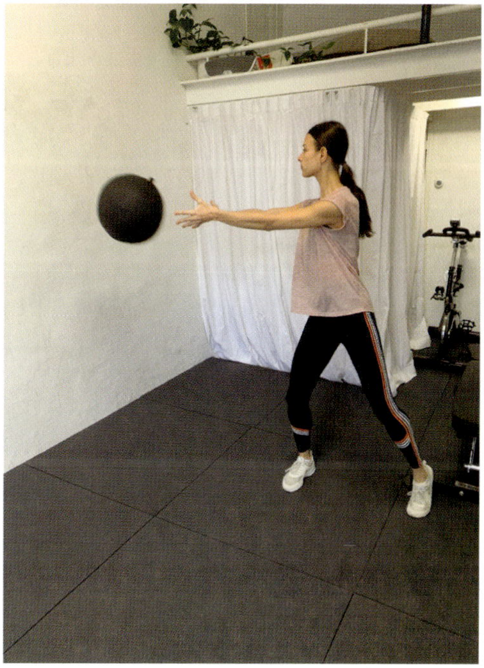

Fig. 212 End position.

PLYOMETRICS

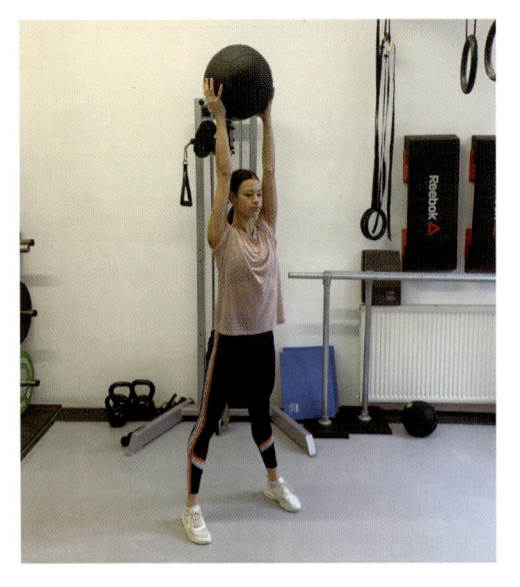

Fig. 213 Medicine ball slam start position.

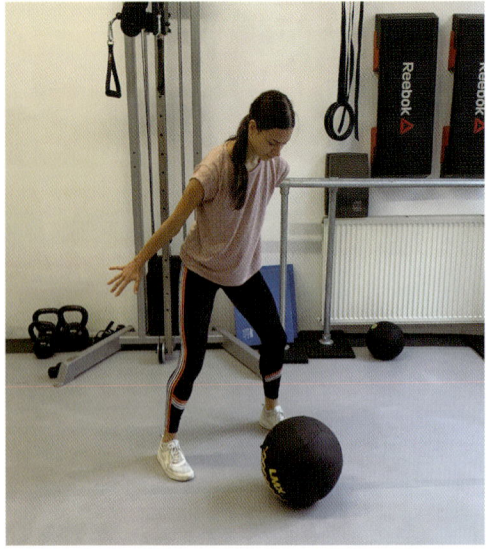

Fig. 214 End position.

3. Your knees and hips should be involved in this movement when performing it (Fig. 216).
4. Be careful to throw the ball away from you so as not to have it come up and hit you.

5. Take the ball and repeat the exercise.
6. This can be done on the same side or in an alternating fashion.
7. It can be performed for time or repetitions.

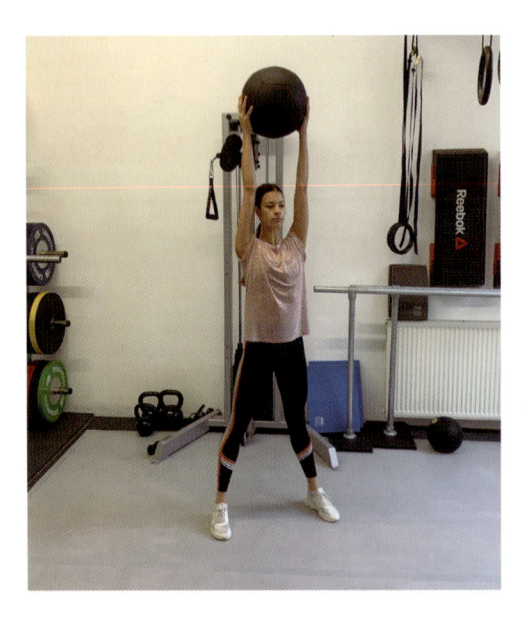

Fig. 215 Medicine ball lateral slam start position.

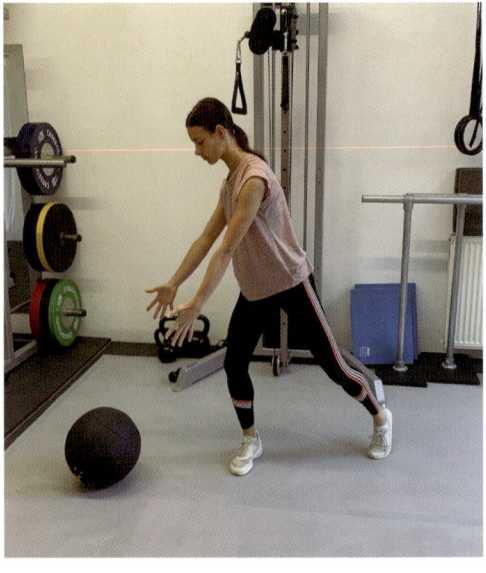

Fig. 216 End position.

PLYOMETRICS

Medicine ball backward throws

For this exercise you will need quite a bit of space, therefore performing it outside is a good option.

1. Hold the medicine ball held in an underhand grip and between your legs.
2. Bend down into a squat position (Fig. 217).
3. Begin by accelerating upwards with your arms, throwing the ball up (Fig. 218) and behind you.
4. You should lift off the ground in a jump and reach what is known as triple extension; there may also be a slight extension of the back as you throw the ball backwards (Fig. 219).
5. Once the ball has landed safely away from you, walk to the ball and repeat the exercise for the required number of repetitions.

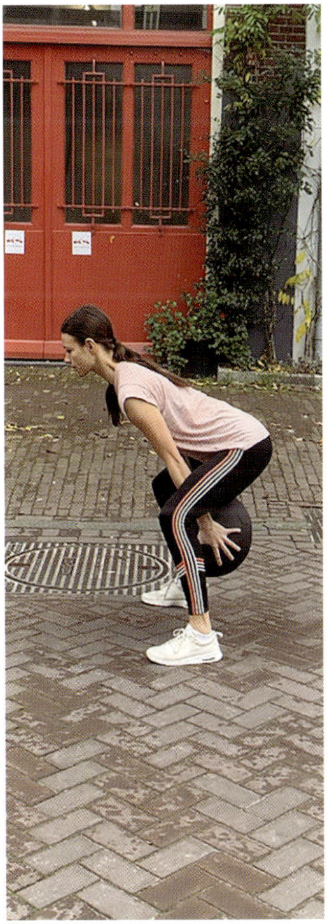

Fig. 217 Medicine ball backward throw start position.

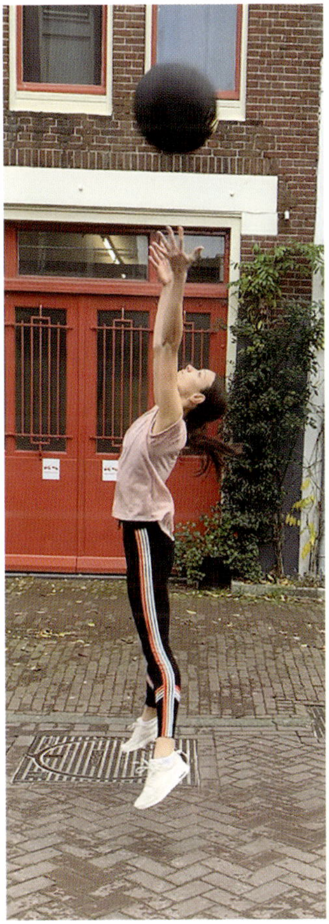

Fig. 218 Mid-movement.

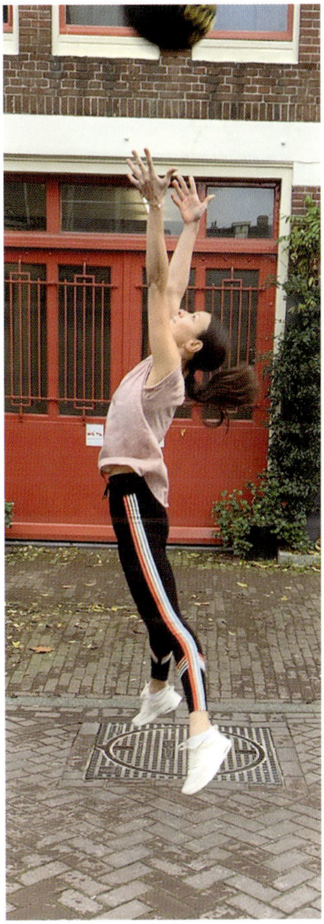

Fig. 219 End position.

10 PROGRAMME IDEAS TO GET YOU STARTED

We have produced six programmes that you can start immediately. These are generic and not specifically designed to your particular needs, but act as a good starting point. There are two programmes each for beginner, intermediate and advanced levels. All of the programmes should be performed twice a week with the appropriate rest days and should not interfere with your training/performance schedule. For example: on a Monday and a Thursday, the whole workout will take you roughly an hour to get through; however, if time is an issue and you find yourself with perhaps 20 to 30 minutes you can split them up into each part separately and do it over six days. An example would look like this:

This way you have still achieved the objective of performing each exercise twice weekly without overloading yourself.

Programme 1		**Programme 4**	
Monday: A1, B1, B2	Friday: C1, C2	Monday: A1, A2	Friday: B1, B2
Tuesday: C1, C2	Saturday: D1, D2	Tuesday: B1, B2	Saturday: C1, C2
Wednesday: D1, D2	Sunday: Rest	Wednesday: C1, C2	Sunday: Rest
Thursday: A1, B1, B2		Thursday: A1, A2	

Table 24 Splitting a programme across multiple days.

PROGRAMME IDEAS TO GET YOU STARTED

Programme Design Explanation

In the programmes you will see a number of headings with variables underneath; these will be explained below.

Order	This dictates how you will perform the exercises chosen.	A1: B1:	Means that you will perform A1 first with the required number of repetitions, sets and rest before moving on to B1.
		A1: A2:	This is known as a paired set meaning that you will perform A1 for the required number of repetitions, rest, then perform A2 for the correct number of reps, rest and then go back and do A1 until you have completed all the sets prescribed.
Exercise	This tells you which exercise is to be performed.		
Repetitions	Within this box it tells you how many reps you must perform and in which week.	8–10 reps	This means you will try to complete 8–10 repetitions of the given exercise.
		8–10/ 7–9/ 6–8/5–7 reps	This means that in week 1 you would try to complete 8–10 reps, in week 2, 7–9 reps, and so on. The drop in repetitions means that the weight must be increased, making the exercise more intense. If you cannot complete the given amount of reps it means the weight is too heavy.
Sets	This tells you how many sets you must perform of the exercise.	3/3/4/4	This means that in weeks 1 and 2 you will perform 3 sets and weeks 3 and 4 you will have to do 4 sets.
Reps in reserve (RIR)	Reps in reserve means how many repetitions you have left in you before technical (form) failure.	2	This means that if you reach your goal of 10 reps but you could have done 4 more the weight is too light, whereas if you could have only achieved 1 more the weight was too heavy.
Rest	This lets you know how much rest in seconds you should take between sets. As you may have noticed, as the intensity of the exercise goes up the rest gets longer. This is because the nature of the exercise is becoming heavier on the nervous system which requires longer rest periods.	60	This refers to 60 seconds' rest between sets.

PROGRAMME IDEAS TO GET YOU STARTED

| Tempo | This lets you know the cadence of the exercise and consists of the time each section of a movement should last. The first digit is the time for the eccentric phase; the second digit is the time in between the eccentric and concentric phases; the third is time for the concentric phase, and the last is the time between repetitions. An 'x' in the tempo box means to perform the exercise as explosively as possible.

NA – means that tempo is not applicable for the exercise. | 3010 | The 3 means you would lower the weight for 3 seconds.

The 0 indicates that there is no pause in the eccentric or stretched position.

The 1 means time it takes for the concentric (flexion) portion of the exercise.

The 0 indicates that there is no pause. |

Table 25 Programme design.

BEGINNER PROGRAMMES

Order	Exercise	Reps: week 1/2/3/4	Sets: week 1/2/3/4	Reps in reserve (RIR)	Rest: week 1/2/3/4	Tempo
A1	Skipping	30 seconds of work	4 sets working up to 10 sets	-	30	-
B1	Front foot elevated split squat	8–10	3	3	60	3010
B2	Incline push-ups	8–10	3	3	60	3010
C1	Swiss ball hamstring curls	8–10	3	3	60	3010
C2	Half-kneeling single arm cable rows	8–10	3	3	60	3010
D1	Kneeling side plank with band	8–10	3	3	60	3010
D2	Deadbugs	16–20 (total)	3	3	60	2020

*Note: start with 4 sets of 30 seconds of skipping and 30 seconds of rest and build up to 10 sets. Once you reach 10 sets, start cutting the rest by 5 seconds every week until you are doing 5 minutes of continuous work.

Table 26 Beginner programme 1.

PROGRAMME IDEAS TO GET YOU STARTED

Order	Exercise	Reps: week 1/2/3/4	Sets: week 1/2/3/4	Reps in reserve (RIR)	Rest: week 1/2/3/4	Tempo
A1	Reverse drop jumps from low step	30 seconds of work	3/3/3/4	2	60–90	-
B1	Lateral step-ups (mid-shin)	8–10	3/3/3/4	2	60	3010
B2	Incline dumbbell press	8–10	3/3/3/4	2	60	3010
C1	Single leg reverse hypers	8–10	3/3/3/4	2	60	3010
C2	Single arm lat pulldowns	8–10	3/3/3/4	2	60	3010
D1	Half kneeling Pallof press	8–10	3	2	60	2020
D2	Bird-dog	16–20 (total)	3	2	60	2020

Table 27 Beginner programme 2.

INTERMEDIATE PROGRAMMES

Order	Exercise	Reps: week 1/2/3/4	Sets: week 1/2/3/4	Reps in reserve (RIR)	Rest: week 1/2/3/4	Tempo
A1	Box jumps	5	4/4/4/4	-	90–120	-
B1	Bulgarian split squats	8–10/7–9/7–9/6–8	3/3/4/4	2	60/75/75/90	3010
B2	Seated dumbbell shoulder press	8–10/7–9/7–9/6–8	3/4/4/4	2	60/75/75/90	3010
C1	Single arm single leg kettlebell deadlift	8–10/7–9/7–9/6–8	3/4/4/4	2	60/75/75/90	3010
C2	Seated cable rows	8–10/7–9/7–9/6–8	3/4/4/4	2	60/75/75/90	3010
D1	Copenhagen side planks	10 second hold × 3–5reps	3	-	60	-

Table 28 Intermediate programme 1.

Order	Exercise	Reps: week 1/2/3/4	Sets: week 1/2/3/4	Reps in reserve (RIR)	Rest: week 1/2/3/4	Tempo
A1	Skater jumps	30 seconds of work	4/4/4/4	-	90	-
A2	Medicine ball slams	10	4/4/4/4	-	90	xxx
B1	Trap bar squat	8–10/7–9/6–8/5–7	3/3/4/4	2	60/75/90/120	3010

PROGRAMME IDEAS TO GET YOU STARTED

B2	Flat dumbbell press	8–10/7–9/ 6–8/5–7	3/3/4/4	2	60/75/90/120	3010
C1	45-degree back extensions	10–12/8–10/ 8–10/7–9	3/3/4/4	2	60/60/60/75	3010
C2	Chest supported dumbbell rows	8–10/7–9/ 6–8/5–7	3/3/4/4	2	60/60/60/75	3010

Table 29 Intermediate programme 2.

ADVANCED PROGRAMMES

Order	Exercise	Reps: week 1/2/3/4	Sets: week 1/2/3/4	Reps in reserve (RIR)	Rest: week 1/2/3/4	Tempo
A1	Medicine ball throws behind	5	4/4/4/4	2	120	-
B1	Sumo deadlift	8–10/7–9/ 6–8/5–7	3/3/4/4	2	90/90/120/120	3010
B2	(Band assisted) chin-ups supinated grip	8–10/7–9/ 6–8/5–7	3/3/4/4	2	90/90/120/120	3010
C1	Standing overhead barbell press	8–10/7–9/ 6–8/5–7	3/3/4/4	2	90/90/120/120	3010
C2	Walking lunges	16–20/ 16–20/ 12–16/12–16	3/3/3/3	2	90/90/120/120	2020

*Note: band assisted is in brackets for those that are not able to achieve the required amount of reps unaided.
**In weeks 3 and 4 the sequence for C1/ C2 is as follows: C1/C2 C1/C2 C1/C2 C1, as there is one more set for upper-body than lower-body.

Table 30 Advanced programme 1.

Order	Exercise	Reps: week 1/2/3/4	Sets: week 1/2/3/4	Reps in reserve (RIR)	Rest: week 1/2/3/4	Tempo
A1	Depth jump with rebound	5	4/4/4/4	-	120	xxxx
A2	Medicine ball oblique toss	10	4/4/4/4	-	120	xxxx
B1	Front squat	6–8/6–8/ 5–7/5–7	3/3/4/4	2	120/120/180/180	3010
B2	Pull-ups	6–8/6–8/ 5–7/5–7	3/3/4/4	2	120/120/180/180	3010
C1	Glute ham raises	6–8/6–8/ 5–7/5–7	3/3/4/4	2	120/120/180/180	3010
C2	Pike push-ups	6–8/6–8/ 5–7/5–7	3/3/4/4	2	120/120/180/180	3010

Table 31 Advanced programme 2.

PROGRAMME IDEAS TO GET YOU STARTED

DEVELOPING YOUR AEROBIC FOUNDATION

The aim is to be able to exercise non-stop at 90 per cent of your heart rate max (Chapter 4) for 30 minutes. Each session should start with a warm-up (4- or 5-minute walk and dynamic stretch) and end with a cooldown (4- or 5-minute walk followed by a stretch, especially of the calves, hamstrings, quads and glutes). The examples below are for developing your running capacity, but they can be transferred to other modes of exercise, with walk corresponding to easy intensity, jog moderate intensity and run high intensity.

Week 1	Jog 2 minutes, walk 1 minute for 20–30 minutes: 3 sessions a week.
Week 2	Jog 3 minutes, walk 1 minute, jog 2 minutes, walk 1 minute, repeat for 20–30 minutes: 4 sessions a week.
Week 3	Jog 3 minutes, walk 1 minute for 20–30 minutes: 4 sessions a week.
Week 4	Jog 5 minutes, walk 1 minute for 20–30 minutes: 4 sessions a week.
Week 5	Jog 5 minutes, walk 1 minute, jog 10 minutes, walk 2 minutes, jog 5 minutes, walk 1 minute, jog 5 minutes, walk 1 minute: 3 sessions a week.
Week 6	Jog 10 minutes, walk 2 minutes × 3: 3 sessions a week.
Week 7	Jog 15 minutes, walk 1 minute, jog 15 minutes: 3 sessions a week.
Week 8	Jog 20–30 minutes: 3 sessions a week.

Table 32 Beginners.

Week 1	Jog 5 minutes, walk 1 minute for 20–30 minutes: 4 sessions a week.
Week 2	Jog 10 minutes, walk 2 minutes × 3: 3 sessions a week.
Week 3	Jog 2 minutes, run 5 minutes, walk 1 minute × 4: 3 sessions a week.
Week 4	Jog 2 minutes, run 5 minutes, jog 2 minutes, run 5 minutes, walk 1 minute × 2: 3 sessions a week.
Week 5	Jog 2 minutes, run 10 minutes, walk 1 minute × 2: 3 sessions a week.
Week 6	Jog 2 minutes, run 15 minutes, jog 2 minutes, walk 1 minute, run 8 minutes, jog 2 minutes: 3 sessions a week.
Week 7	Jog 2 minutes, run 20 minutes, jog 1 minute, run 8 minutes: 3 sessions a week.
Week 8	Jog 2 minutes, run 25–30 minutes: 3 sessions a week.

Table 33 Intermediate.

Week 1	Jog 2 minutes, run 5 minutes, jog 2 minutes, run 5 minutes, walk 1 minute × 2: 3 sessions a week.
Week 2	Jog 2 minutes, run 15 minutes, jog 1 minutes, run 15 minutes, jog 2 minutes: 3 sessions a week.
Week 3	Jog 2 minutes, run 25–30 minutes: 3 sessions a week.
Week 4	Jog 2 minutes, run 25–30 minutes: 3 sessions a week.
Week 5	Jog 2 minutes, run 25–30 minutes: 3 sessions a week.
Week 6	Jog 2 minutes, run 25–30 minutes: 3 sessions a week.

Table 34 Advanced.

PROGRAMME IDEAS TO GET YOU STARTED

Circuit training

Although circuit training is often classified as HIIT, it doesn't really meet the criteria as heart rates remain high and constant throughout. It has been shown to develop aerobic fitness and local muscular endurance. There are no ideal formats for the sequence of circuit exercises, but the general principles should not be to tax any one particular muscle too much, so that local fatigue doesn't mean a drop in intensity.

Circuit 1	Circuit 2
Each exercise for 1 minute	20 reps of exercise and 2 minutes skipping
Press-ups	Press-ups
Calf raises	Squats
Skipping	Crunches
Bicep curls with Dynaband or hand weights	Skipping
Crunches	Seated row (Dynaband around feet, legs straight, pull hands to hips)
Skipping	Lunges
Bench dips	Toe touches
Plank	Skipping
Skipping	Upright row with Dynaband or hand weights
Straight leg bows (keep legs straight – bend from waist and grip near feet – straighten until upright, pulling on band)	Tuck jumps
	Plank
	Skipping
Toe touch sit-ups	Bench dips
Skipping	Calf raises
Pull-ups (under bar or using edge of a table)	Side plank
Side plank	Skipping
Skipping	Bicep curl with Dynaband or hand weights
Upright row with Dynaband or hand weights	Triceps overhead extension with Dynaband or hand weights
Reverse curl	Ball pikes
Skipping	Skipping
Hamstring curls with Swiss ball	
Hyperextensions	
Skipping	

Table 35 Circuit training.

PROGRAMME IDEAS TO GET YOU STARTED

HIGH INTENSITY INTERVAL TRAINING (HIIT)

Aerobic

The format for aerobic interval training is 2–3 minutes of hard exercise followed by 2–3 minutes of recovery exercise. As noted in Chapter 4, you need to have a good aerobic foundation, as this will help your recovery between hard sets. During the hard exercise periods you need to push yourself as hard as possible. Total exercise time doesn't need to be more than 30 minutes. An adaptation of the DAFT can be used as a dance movement alternative to running, cycling or cross trainer.

Time	Tempo	Movement
2 min	108	5 springs, lunge and recover. 3 spring hops in a circle, include arm movements. 4 sets of hop, hop with 90° turn between each set, arms moving between first and second position.
2 min	easy	Walk recovery.
2 min	108	5 springs, lunge and recover. 3 spring hops in a circle, include arm movements. 4 sets of hop, hop with 90° turn between each set, arms moving between first and second position.
2 min	easy	Walk recovery.

Table 36 HIIT training.

Anaerobic

This is really hard training as it targets the anaerobic system. You need to exercise as hard as you can for 60–90 seconds before recovering for 180–270 seconds; it looks easier than the aerobic intervals, but the exercise period must be much, much harder. To reach the required intensities the simpler the exercise you do the better: running, rowing, cross-trainer are ideal but you can use a dance version as well. You can adapt the high-intensity dance performance test into a training format. Total training time is around 20–30 minutes.

It isn't enjoyable but is essential, as this system is rarely used outside of dance performance. The joy comes 30–60 minutes after the session when you have realized you are still alive.

Time	Tempo	Movement
1 min	106	4 sets of 2 jumps with 90° jump turn between each set, arms moving between first and fifth position; 2 springs forwards, roll to floor touching the back, 2 steps out into a lunge with a 180° turn to face direction you've come from; big 2-footed jump forwards with arms, mini-handstand, run backwards, star steps. Start phrase on left.
3 min		Recovery.
1 min	106	Repeat first stage but starting on right.

Table 37 Anaerobic training.

11 | DANCE NUTRITION

by Tommy Zarate

Introduction

The foods we eat not only supply our body with the energy we need for the activities of daily life and intense training, but can also positively (and negatively) affect our mood, growth, immune system, and hormones. Strategically implemented, sports nutrition can also increase performance and promote recovery and regeneration. In this chapter, we will briefly discuss the fundamentals of nutrition and how to implement a sports nutritional strategy. Finally, we will discuss an emerging 'hot topic' known as relative energy deficiency in sport (RED-S).

Digestion and absorption

It is important to understand what takes place before we can extract the energy from food and subsequently use that energy to fuel training and performance. Digestion starts at the mouth but involves many organs. When we eat, digestion occurs in the form of mechanical and chemical digestion. While both happen at the same time, they work in very distinct ways. Mechanical digestion breaks larger pieces of food into smaller pieces via chewing and mixing. This helps increase the efficiency of chemical digestion. As food passes from the mouth to the stomach, various gastric juices and peristalsis (the mixing) in the stomach begin turning food into a liquid or paste called chyme. Emptying of the stomach usually takes 2–6 hours.

Once food leaves the stomach it enters the small intestine, where partially digested nutrients are further broken down and absorption occurs. Roughly 95 per cent of absorption occurs in the small intestine and that's due to its design. The lumen of the small intestine is not flat: there are large folds, finger-like projections, and hair-like extensions called Kerckring folds, villi, and microvilli, respectively. These structures help increase the surface area of the small intestine to roughly 30–40 m^2 – half of a badminton court. Here, proteins, carbohydrates, and fats will be absorbed, subsequently being released into the blood stream or lymphatic system where they will end up passing through the liver before being released to target cells throughout the body. Any food matter that escapes absorption is fermented in the large intestine or excreted.

Calories, energy balance, and energy expenditure

Let's first define a few terms. A calorie is a measurement of energy. A single calorie is required to raise the temperature of 1g of water by 1° Celsius. In nutrition, however, the word 'calorie' refers to kilocalories (kcal), or 1,000 calories. Additionally, depending on where you are in the world, you might see kilojoules on a nutrition label. For reference, 1 kilocalorie is equal to 4.18 kilojoules, but moving forward, we will simply refer to energy in kilocalories.

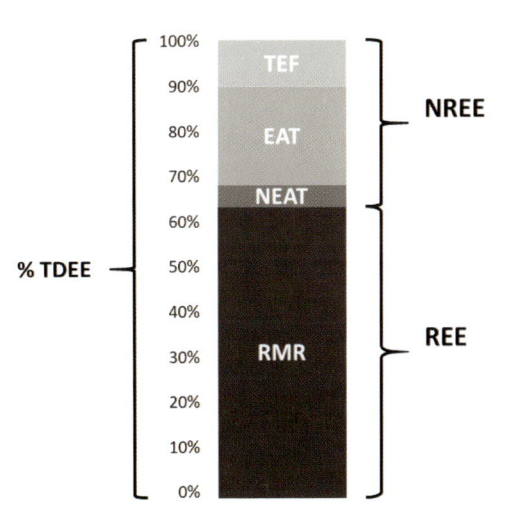

Total daily energy expenditure (TDEE) can be divided into unique categories (Fig. 220). These categories include:

- **Resting metabolic rate (RMR):** the energy required to maintain normal body functions and homeostasis. In inactive populations, this normally accounts for 60–75 per cent of total energy expenditure. The amount of energy (kcal) expended is largely related to bodyweight, age, gender, and body composition.
- **Non-exercise activity thermogenesis (NEAT):** this represents the energy expenditure during daily activity without including exercise. This can include walking, gardening, fidgeting, and shivering when you're cold.
- **Exercise activity thermogenesis (EAT), or thermic effect of exercise:** this is the most variable component of total daily energy expenditure and includes training, exercise, and competition. This has been shown to range between 30 per cent and 80 per cent of TDEE and depends on the duration and type of activity an athlete is involved in.
- **Diet-induced thermogenesis (TEF):** this accounts for the amount of energy needed to digest, absorb, transport, and store nutrients. This varies depending on the composition of your diet; however, it

Fig. 220 Total daily energy expenditure (%).

generally makes up ~10 per cent of total daily energy expenditure.

When an athlete is weight-stable over a period of time, they are considered to be in a state of 'energy balance'. This suggests that the amount of energy being expended is equally met by food intake; calories out = calories in. Ironically, we're very briefly in a state of true energy balance. Within a 24-hour period, energy balance is constantly changing. For example, after waking from an overnight fast and before any food is consumed, an individual will be in a negative energy balance (i.e. they will be expending more calories than they are supplying). Consuming a meal and shortly after, the individual will now be in a positive energy balance. This is generally followed by a short fasting period – between meals – in which the cycle will repeat itself. When attempting to manipulate body mass, it is important to impose an energy deficit or surplus over an appropriate period of time. The body has multiple ways to compensate for any changes to energy balance, such as subconsciously decreasing or increasing non-exercise activity, increasing appetite and hunger, or increasing metabolic rate.

DANCE NUTRITION

In a cohort of fifty ballet, jazz, and contemporary dance students, total daily energy expenditure was shown to be ~3,400 and ~2,250 kcal for men and women, respectively. During dance sessions, energy expenditure was estimated to be around 330 calories for all three disciplines. These values were somewhat similar to both pre-professional contemporary and elite ballet female dancers.

MACRONUTRIENTS AND MICRONUTRIENTS FOR DANCERS

The food we consume provides the body with nutrients and these nutrients are divided into six categories: protein, fat, carbohydrates, water, vitamins, and minerals. Nutrients do more than provide fuel for the body: they also promote growth and repair and regulate metabolism. Macro- and micro- refer to the amount of these nutrients required by the body. Macronutrients require much more than 1g per day and micronutrients require roughly 1g per day.

Protein

Amino acids are the building blocks of protein. Out of the twenty amino acids found in dietary protein, nine are considered essential (EAA) and the remaining eleven are non-essential (NEAA). Essential amino acids cannot be synthesized in the body; therefore, they must be obtained through food consumption. The other eleven amino acids can be manufactured and obtained from the amino acid pool or by recycling amino acids from protein breakdown. Every cell in the human body uses protein as a structure and proteins are integral components of cell membranes, and the development of peptide hormones and enzymes. Protein also has the highest dietary-induced thermogenesis and plays a key role in body composition change. The most common association of protein within the body is skeletal muscle; skin, hair, and nails are also largely composed of protein. Key benefits of eating adequate protein include increased strength, muscle mass, and minimizing muscle tissue during weight loss.

The quality of a protein source depends on the composition of amino acids within a food or food product. A high-quality source of protein (complete protein) will contain all nine essential amino acids, whereas a low-quality protein (incomplete protein) lacks a sufficient amount of one or more essential amino acids. Dietary proteins are derived from

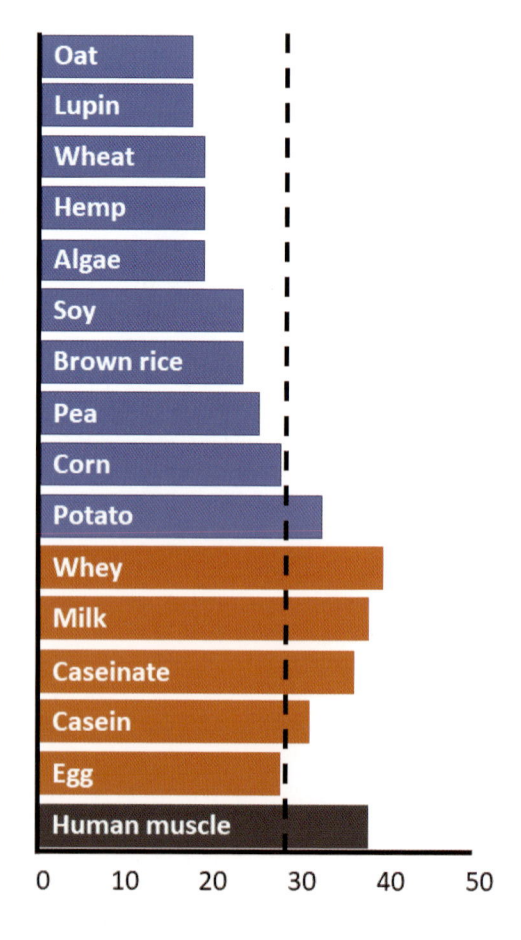

Fig. 221 Essential amino acids as percentage of total protein.

DANCE NUTRITION

animal-based and plant-based food products. Examples of animal-based protein sources include meat, poultry, eggs, fish, and some dairy products. Plant-based sources include whole grains, legumes, and some vegetable products. Because grains and legumes lack lysine and methionine, respectively, they are considered incomplete proteins. It is therefore recommended that athletes with a plant-based diet consume more than one source of protein per meal.

The recommended daily allowance (RDA) for protein is 0.8 grams per kilogram (g/kg) of bodyweight. For example, a 70kg individual should aim to consume 56g of protein per day. This could be met by consuming 57g of smoked salmon, 1 wholewheat bagel, 3 whole eggs, and 65g of Greek yoghurt. As an athlete, it is imperative to understand that the RDA for protein may not be enough to support the desired training adaptations (e.g. building muscle). The American College of Sports Medicine's position on dietary practices for athletes recommends protein intake upwards of 1.2–1.7 g/kg of bodyweight to support the repair, regeneration, and synthesis of new body tissues. The increase in dietary protein needs is easily met without the use of supplementation. In addition to the sample intake above, an athlete would only need to include 125g of canned beans, 65g of quinoa, 1 skinless, boneless chicken thigh, and 125ml of milk to meet the needs of training. Special consideration should be given to the amount of protein and leucine, an EAA, consumed in a single meal. Leucine is known to be a potent stimulator of muscle protein synthesis (MPS) and without a sufficient protein feeding, maximizing MPS will require a larger protein feeding (i.e. you will need to eat more protein for the desired effect).

Protein plays a large role in maintaining a properly functioning body; however, healthy athletes void of any unmanaged clinical pathologies should focus on maintaining an optimal body composition and performance. Due to the body's inability to synthesize essential amino acids, protein consumption is important for manufacturing and repair of muscle and other body tissues. Animal-based products are considered high-quality protein; however, this shouldn't discount the intake of plant-based protein sources in an athlete's diet. When plant sources of amino acids are combined (e.g. beans and quinoa) with or without animal sources, each source becomes complementary and enables an athlete to meet dietary requirements to optimize athletic performance, health and well-being.

Carbohydrate

Carbohydrates, also known as saccharides, provide energy during physical activity and are a critical component to the athlete's diet. Carbohydrates can be stored in the liver, muscle, to a very small extent in the kidneys, and are also circulating in blood. Glucose derived from carbohydrates is used in muscle tissue, the brain, and also red blood cells. Dance of various styles requires repeated bouts of high-intensity muscle contractions and endurance. Running, jumping, high-velocity transitions and static holds are regular movements in dance performance. Hard and high-intensity training should be matched with food products rich in carbohydrates to maintain training intensity during prolonged training sessions and to maintain day-to-day performance. Suboptimal carbohydrate intake can lead to an undesired reduction in intensity and may lead to increased sickness, injury, and exacerbate negative changes in mood.

Rich sources of carbohydrates are found in fruits, some vegetables, breads, grains, and pasta. Desserts, cakes, pastries, and candy can also provide a rich source of carbohydrates, but these food items may lack key nutrients (e.g. vitamins and minerals) and contain higher amounts of saturated fat due to ultra-processing. While there are multiple types of carbohydrates, glucose, fructose, sucrose, and starch are the most prevalent sources found in the diet. Once a saccharide enters the liver, it is ultimately converted into glucose for storage, oxidation, or transported to peripheral tissue. Carbohydrate availability refers to the amount of carbohydrate included in a food or food product per serving. Generally, foods with high carbohydrate availability will be low in fibre and protein and low-to-moderate in water content, such as white bread, pasta, and rice. Foods with low carbohydrate availability include beans (which contain a moderate amount of fibre and protein) or watermelon (high in water content).

Muscle glycogen

This is the most important substrate for training and competition because it can be broken down and used for energy quickly. When the demand for energy is very high, glycogen is broken down anaerobically and when exercise intensity is moderate-to-high, glycogen can be oxidized aerobically. It is important to know that these two metabolic processes occur at the same time, but the contribution depends on intensity and duration of exercise. Roughly 300–600g of glucose can be stored within skeletal muscle in trained athletes.

Liver glycogen

Liver glycogen, on the other hand, is important for maintaining blood glucose levels and the prevention of hypoglycaemia (low blood sugar). Symptoms of hypoglycaemia include, but are not limited to, loss of motor skill, dizziness, disorientation, and cold sweats and this is detrimental to dance performance. In athletes with diabetes mellitus, this can be fatal. The liver has a higher concentration of glycogen than muscle; however, due to its size, roughly only 80–110g of glucose can be stored.

Below, we will discuss carbohydrate intake in relation to the training and competition or performance schedule.

In the months and weeks leading up to a competition: carbohydrate needs are largely dictated by training intensity and duration. Because glycogen stores can be completely depleted after training, restoring glycogen stores becomes an important daily task so that subsequent training session performance (e.g. on the same or next day) can be maintained. Daily carbohydrate intake ranges from 3–5g/kg of bodyweight per day during low-to-moderate intensity and technical training days. This can be accomplished by consuming nutrient-rich carbohydrates sources at each meal. Carbohydrate sources during this

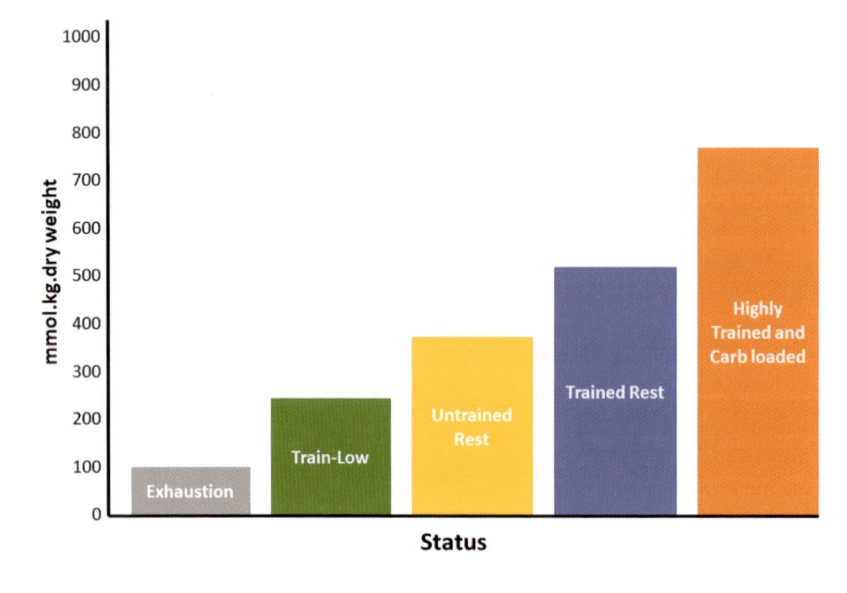

Fig. 222 Muscle glycogen content according to training status.

period include whole grains and wheat bread, muesli, quinoa, couscous, fruits and vegetables. While it is encouraged to replace lost carbohydrate stores following training, training demand may not completely exhaust glycogen stores and ensuring total daily carbohydrate intake requirements will be sufficient.

For a 70kg dancer to meet daily requirements of 3–5g/kg of bodyweight, they would need to consume:

- 1 wholewheat bagel and 1 banana for breakfast
- 190g of brown rice and 30g of dried fruit for lunch
- An apple and granola bar around training
- 1 serving of wheat pasta for dinner with a serving of ice cream for dessert

Research investigating nutritional intake in dancers remains scarce, but there are reasonable justifications for a carbohydrate intake of up to 5–7g/kg of bodyweight per day. The addition of a strength and conditioning programme, and an increase in training duration, or frequency, are all valid reasons. These recommendations can be met by increasing an individual's number of servings or serving sizes of carbohydrate-rich foods, in addition to diligently refuelling in the 'post-training window'. Any delay in food consumption reduces the time available for refuelling. For athletes who have difficulty consuming large quantities of food, switching to foods with high carbohydrate availability during this period can be effective – and more importantly very enjoyable. Some practical recommendations include switching to white bread, rice, and pasta, and including fresh fruit juice. Be aware that a short-term increase in carbohydrate intake may cause an increase in bodyweight; however, this increase is likely due to an increase in water weight and not fat. Consulting with a qualified sports nutritionist or dietitian at this point is recommended for a comprehensive assessment of training demand and nutritional intake. Any mismatch in energy output or energy input may lead to suboptimal performance or may negatively impact body composition.

In the days leading up to a performance: it is important to maintain carbohydrate intake at the level of training. More importantly, carbohydrate intake should not be completely omitted from the diet. However, if training demand remains relatively stable and no taper has occurred, maintaining carbohydrate intake may be beneficial.

With 24 hours or less until performance: switching carbohydrate sources to easily digestible food and food products can be an effective strategy. This may help with body appearance and costume aesthetics and muscle glycogen storage.

In the 3 to 5 hours prior to performance: the athlete should continue to focus on easily digestible, high carbohydrate available food sources. Familiar foods will help minimize any unnecessary GI issues, and the high carbohydrate available foods will top-up muscle and liver glycogen stores. This time period is absolutely critical for any competitive dancer. Without this top-up, dancers run the risk of premature muscle fatigue and subpar performances. It is also worth considering any pre-competition nerves. Dancers may experience anxiety and/or stress that decreases appetite, so a practical approach should be developed beforehand.

In the 3–5 hours prior to show time, a 60kg dancer can consume two carbohydrate-rich meals, consisting of, for example:

- (earlier meal) a bowl of porridge with skimmed milk, 1 apple with a tablespoon of peanut butter, and a glass of fruit juice
- (meal closer to performance) 3 slices of white toast with jam and a can of their preferred soft drink

This is approximately 175g of carbohydrates that should be adjusted to fit the needs of each individual dancer depending on body size and performance duration.

In the 1 to 2 hours leading into a performance: dancers need to be strategic with their food consumption. The meals consumed earlier in the day should be enough to maintain glycogen stores; however, a miscalculated approach shortly before competition can be detrimental to physical or mental performance, aesthetics, or cause GI complications. Also, performance days are often very busy and leave little time for other tasks, and venues may not provide any food or food products. Therefore, dancers are encouraged to take initiative and bring a variety of familiar snacks with them to manage any lingering hunger and to supply the body with additional carbohydrate.

Maintaining muscle and liver glycogen is crucial for the professional dancer and the post-exercise window presents a great opportunity for restoration. A variety of different carbohydrate sources are available, and their intake is largely dependent on the time between training sessions, personal preference, and the desired training adaptation. Therefore, including carbohydrates at differing levels (fuelling for the work required) with meals throughout the day is a winning strategy. It is important to know that when glycogen stores are completely exhausted, complete restoration in the meal following training may not be possible. When time between training sessions is long (>12 hours), a combination of foods with high- and low-carbohydrate availability is recommended. However, when the period between training sessions is short (<4 hours), low-fibre, high-carbohydrate sources are recommended. When carbohydrates in the form of whole foods aren't available or appealing, liquid sources of carbohydrates can help replace glycogen and are also perfect for rehydration.

Fat

Dietary fat performs many roles in the body. It assists fat-soluble vitamin transport, is a crucial component of cell membranes and organelles, provides energy, and also gives food a more pleasant texture and aroma. Foods rich in fat content include nuts, seeds, oils, fatty cuts of meat, and some dairy products such as cream and butter. Unlike carbohydrates and protein, fat contains 9kcal/g. Fat in the body exists in various forms and these are classified as different types of lipids. For example, energy is derived from simple lipids, such as triacylglycerols, and cholesterol is an example of a derived lipid. Fats can also be categorized as saturated or unsaturated. Triacylglycerols are the most abundant dietary lipid consumed and are the main source of energy for use during exercise and at rest.

Fat tissue also protects major organs and is a precursor for steroid hormones. It is suggested that essential fatty acids aid in health promotion and performance, while excessive consumption of certain fats has been linked to high cholesterol, LDL, or certain cancers. Expert sources suggest that saturated fat and trans-fat should make up <10% and <1% of total fat intake respectively.

During exercise, adipose tissue and muscle tissue use fatty acids to create energy. Compared to glycogen, lipids can store up to fifty times more energy. This highlights the importance of fat as a fuel source during endurance and prolonged exercise. As exercise duration increases, fat use increases, and glycogen use decreases. In a metabolically healthy dancer, fat use is the preferred source of energy at rest, during low-intensity exercise, and even moderate-intensity exercise in well-trained athletes. Fat as a fuel fails during very-high-intensity exercise because the rate of fat breakdown cannot supply energy fast enough to accommodate the demand for ATP (the body's energy currency). Remember, anaerobic metabolism uses only glucose.

DANCE NUTRITION

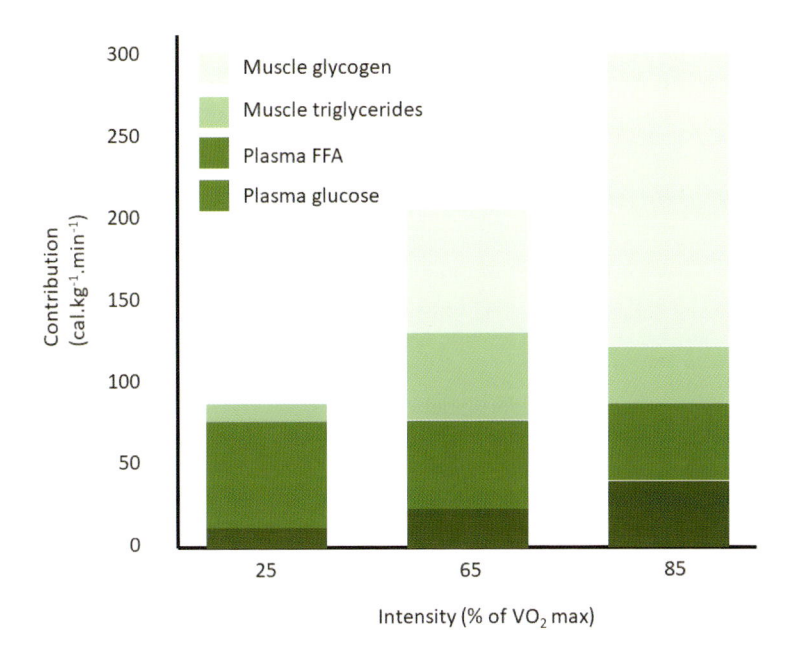

Fig. 223 Energy source for exercise at different intensities.

Attempting to increase performance by eating a high fat diet prior to exercise may lead to increased fat use but benefits to performance have not been seen. This approach may be applicable for a recreational dancer, but not for competitive and elite dancers. There's no evidence to suggest a high-fat diet other than personal preference. Other methods for increasing fat use during exercise include fasting, low-carbohydrate diets, and also the Ketogenic diet. These approaches do increase fat use, but limiting carbohydrates leads to decreased performance at higher intensities. When exercise intensity is low (~45% VO$_2$max), fasted training doesn't affect performance; however, performance is affected when training intensity increases, or the fasting period increases (>12 hours). The main mechanisms haven't been identified, but liver glycogen depletion could be a factor. The Ketogenic diet is an extreme low-carbohydrate/high-fat diet. When you restrict carbohydrate and increase fat intake, the liver creates ketone bodies (ketogenesis) for energy. Most organs can use ketones as a fuel source, but unsurprisingly, this increase in ketone use doesn't translate to increased performance. There have also been reports of high-fat meals causing GI disturbances prior to exercise.

Omega–3 essential fatty acids have shown promise as an ergogenic aid in athletes. Because essential fatty acids cannot be created in the body, they must be consumed through certain foods and food products. These food sources include nuts, seeds, oils, algae, and fatty fish. Eicosapentaenoic acid (EPA) and docosahexaenoic acid (DHA) are polyunsaturated fatty acids and can be found in cold-water fish such as sardines, salmon, tuna, algae, and krill. Plant sources of omega–3s include flaxseed, canola oil, and some nuts and seeds; however, plant-based foods are not good sources for EPA or DHA. The conversion of plant-based Omega–3 to EPA and DHA are very low; roughly 1–10 per cent. Supplements are also available as different fish- and plant-based oils. In athletes, EPA and DHA supplementation have been shown to increase various strength and endurance parameters, as well as reduce exercise-induced fatigue. Many of these performance benefits are normally seen after chronic supplementation (>4 weeks). Controversy surrounds the true effectiveness of omega–3 supplementation for performance and benefits may only be seen when the omega–3 fatty acid index improves from suboptimal to optimal. This means that any increase from optimal likely does not equal better performance.

Hydration and fluid intake

The body is composed of roughly 60 per cent water in healthy adults. Two-thirds of total body water is located inside our cells and the remaining one-third is circulating in plasma and interstitial fluid. Optimal water balance is called euhydration. Dehydration is the process of losing water and when the body is dehydrated, or hypohydrated, athletic performance and cognitive function decrease. When muscle contracts, heat is created. When core temperature increases, thermoreceptors signal the brain to manage this heat by increasing blood flow to the skin and initiate sweating. Therefore, starting exercise with good hydration is key for performance.

Dehydration during exercise is a contributing factor to performance loss. It has been suggested that just a 2 per cent loss in body mass can impair cardiovascular function and any increases in fluid loss continue to negatively affect exercise and performance. Dehydration causes a decrease in blood volume and sweat rate, leading to a decrease in thermoregulation, and also increases the rate of muscle glycogen. This can be avoided by creating a plan that emphasizes starting exercise in a hydrated state, consuming fluids during exercise, and replacing fluids after exercise. A plan is essential for competitive and recreational dancers looking for an edge over their competition.

Recommended intake for healthy adults ranges from 2–2.7 litres per day and 2.5–3.7 litres per day, in females and males, respectively. However, this does not account for fluid loss through exercise. Urine colour can be used to estimate hydration status. Pale yellow generally indicates euhydration, while a darker urine colour indicates hypohydration. Be aware that some supplements (e.g. B vitamins) can change urine colour. Before exercise, 500ml of fluids should be consumed two hours before training and another 500ml consumed fifteen minutes prior to beginning exercise. To individualize a pre-exercise hydration strategy even further, 6–8ml of fluids per kilogram of bodyweight is a great starting point. For a 75kg athlete, this equates to 450–600ml of fluids.

During exercise, fluids should be consumed at regular intervals (e.g. every 15–30 minutes) to prevent weight loss of greater than 2 per cent bodyweight (1.2kg in a 60kg athlete). The amount and frequency of fluid intake in hot and humid conditions should be increased and cooler water temperature may be beneficial. Athletes should be aware that excessive hyperhydrating may not be ideal during exercise. This can negatively affect performance by causing GI issues, unnecessary weight gain, or hyponatremia. Slower athletes or athletes engaged in very low-intensity training can experiment with drinking to thirst; however, when performance and intensity are high, drinking at regular intervals is advised. Some situations in dance prohibit the consumption of solid food during breaks, possibly due to lack of time or fear of GI discomfort. In the case of intense exercise lasting over 60 minutes, a sports drink may be appropriate to replenish liver glycogen stores and to aid in rehydration.

Following exercise, it is recommended that athletes replace 125–150 per cent of total bodyweight lost within an hour. If an 80kg dancer loses 1.5kg during exercise, they should consume 1.9–2.3 litres. This takes into account the additional sweat lost post-exercise and the fluids lost through urination after rehydration. Rehydration can come from water; however, other beverages can be effective. Chocolate milk, for example, contains electrolytes, protein, carbohydrates, and other nutrients. These nutrients aid in recovery, the restoration of glycogen, and also assist fluid retention. The post-rehydration period should also be seen as restoring euhydration for the next training session.

Micronutrients for dance

Micronutrients aid in metabolism, promoting growth and development, and are also involved in creating specific cells and tissues. Their consumption is only required in small quantities and can be found in various foods. Some vitamins can be synthesized in the body but nearly all micronutrients must be acquired by consuming a balanced diet of various foods. Micronutrients can be classified as water-soluble and fat-soluble vitamins, and minerals. Water-soluble vitamins cannot be stored in the body for long periods of time like fat-soluble vitamins can be. Storage of water-soluble vitamins happen because they bind to certain proteins and enzymes, trapping them within a cell. Fat-soluble vitamins, on the other hand, are stored in lipids. Two common micronutrient deficiencies that have been shown to affect exercise and sports performance are vitamin D and iron.

Vitamin D

This fat-soluble vitamin acts similar to a pro-hormone because its precursor transforms into active metabolites. It plays an active role in immune, muscle and cardiovascular function, protein synthesis, and cell growth. Vitamin D can be found in liver, fatty fish, and fortified foods such as milk, orange juice, and cereals. These foods are generally low in vitamin D content or are not effectively converted to vitamin D's active metabolite. UVB from sun exposure and supplementation are better sources of vitamin D3. Geographical location affects UVB exposure with higher latitudes being shown to have less exposure to UVB, especially in the winter months. Because dancers spend most of their time training indoors and away from sun exposure, vitamin D deficiency has been found. If your blood serum vitamin D status is optimal, increasing concentration probably won't provide added benefit. However, if you are deficient, increasing serum concentrations can improve muscle function, recovery time, and decrease injury and illness frequency. Vitamin D is also essential for bone growth, density, and remodelling.

Iron

Iron is essential for the synthesis and functioning of haemoglobin and myoglobin – oxygen carrying proteins. This allows oxygen to be delivered to muscle tissue. Cytochromes in the electron transport chain (ETC) also contain iron and transport oxygen and electrons to create ATP. Iron deficiency has three distinct stages – iron depleted, iron deficient, and iron deficiency with anaemia – which are more common in female athletes. While the iron-depleted state may not generally lead to performance reductions, the latter stages have been shown to decrease oxygen uptake and endurance performance and increase infections. The main cause of iron deficiency is the lack of consuming iron-rich foods. Food that contains iron can be categorized as haem-iron, which has high bioavailability, or non-haem iron, which has low bioavailability. The former comes mainly from animal-based products such as meat, fish, and poultry, while the latter comes from plant- and dairy-based foods. The RDA for iron in adults aged nineteen to fifty years old is 8mg and 18mg for males and females, respectively.

In order for our body to use food as fuel and to provide substrates for its many functions, digestion must effectively and efficiently break food down and prepare the constituents for absorption. Here, they will travel through the intestine, into the lymphatic system or bloodstream, and finally to the liver. Fats, proteins, and carbohydrates are then used for energy, stored for later use, or incorporated into proteins. Protein is essential for muscle growth, retention and repair, while fat and carbohydrate provide the energy needed during strength and conditioning and dance training.

Micronutrients extracted from food are essential for normal growth, energy production, and are used as co-factors for metabolism. In addition, water, the fourth macronutrient, maintains fluid volume in the various compartments, mitigates thermal stress and facilitates performance. Neglecting food intake prior or after training and competition can lead to poor performance and failure to properly fuel the next training session – highlighting the implications of nutrient timing for performance.

Relative Energy Deficiency in Sport (RED-S)

In sports promoting a certain body image, aesthetics, and perfectionism, disordered eating is commonly seen. A 2013 systematic review and meta-analysis reported that the prevalence of eating disorders in female dancers was 12 per cent, and 16.4 per cent in ballet dancers alone. It also suggested that ballet dancers were twice as likely to develop an eating disorder compared to non-dancers. The drive for the perfect body composition, in addition to overtraining, can have negative physiological effects. Male dancers, who are unsurprisingly subjected to the pressures of maintaining a strong and lean physique, have also been shown to exhibit symptoms of disordered eating and body composition concerns. Constant and unnecessary pressures can manifest in undereating, leading to low-energy availability (LEA) and the development of relative energy deficiency in sport (RED-S). LEA is the mismatch of food consumption and the energy needed to maintain performance and health. This condition negatively affects many systems of the body.

RED-S affects exercise performance indirectly by reducing recovery and impairing muscle function. This reduction in food intake leaves the body without the substrates needed to repair and remodel muscle tissue and replenish glycogen stores. Additionally, impaired immune function and the risk of injury are also increased by low energy availability – leading to a loss of training time. LEA also exerts negative effects on the endocrine system which can be detrimental to an athlete's health, affecting metabolic rate and bone. For example, although weight-bearing exercise has been shown to promote the formation and maintenance of bone, reduced energy availability blunts this effect in the short- and long-term. In the short-term, LEA negatively affects bone metabolism by increasing bone resorption markers and decreasing bone formation markers. The lower the energy availability, the larger the effects. Long-term LEA, on the other hand, suppresses hormonal pathways involved in bone metabolism. In females, the suppression of these hormones leads to a loss in menstrual function which has been associated with reduced bone mass and an increase in stress fracture incidence. While male athletes may be more resistant, the effects of LEA on bone mineral density have been shown in endurance-trained males, and in male athletes in sports that require constant or repeated weight loss.

An unexpected factor in the development of RED-S is the influence of the dancer's support team. Unknowingly, coaches, teammates, and family members, can make inappropriate comments about an athlete's body image causing psychological stress, or promote ill-informed training and nutrition recommendations (e.g. 'no days-off' and diuretic use). Many of these concerns can be mitigated by working with the proper healthcare professionals and subject matter experts, who can offer support and provide evidence-based recommendations. The media, including social media, present another set of uncontrollable problems. With the increase in reach and anonymity, social media 'trolls' at all levels have the platform to make shameful and completely unsolicited remarks about people in the media. These comments tend not to go unseen and can sometimes go viral, especially within an athlete's circle.

The management of RED-S requires routine screening, increased awareness, and education, and knowing which populations are high-risk. While it may seem easy to rest and eat more, it is unknown how long the effects of RED-S may last; therefore treatment must be handled by medical professionals. Many tools are available for screening, such as the Relative Energy Deficiency in Sport Clinical Assessment Tool (RED-S CAT), the Low-Energy Availability in Females Questionnaire (LEAF-Q), validated eating disorder questionnaires, and also routine health checks conducted by members of medical staff. While many tools for the management and treatment of RED-S/LEA must be done by the appropriate medical staff, team members can help by making the athletic environment feel like a safe space. Bringing awareness to the severity of the condition, educating athletes on proper nutrition and training principles, and starting the conversation early are all practical recommendations.

Relative energy deficiency in sport is a condition characterized by low-energy availability found in both male and female athletes. Pressure from the media, teammates, and self, contribute to the constant and viscous weight-cycling and the manipulation of body composition in an effort for aesthetics. Compounded by periods of non-functional overtraining, the consequences from RED-S include both physiological and psychological stress. Educating athletes, coaches, and staff members is necessary for preventing RED-S and identifying its signs and symptoms.

SUPPLEMENTS AND ERGOGENIC AIDS

The sports nutrition and dietary supplement market generated over £15bn in 2019, up from £12bn in 2015. Protein supplements alone dominated the market, accounting for over 80 per cent of generated income. Supplement use in the general population is reported to be over 70 per cent, and in 2019, over 80 per cent of youth athletes, aged 15–18, consumed supplements. Motivations for consuming supplements include maintaining or improving health, enhancing physical and mental performance, or manipulating body composition. While there are claims for supplement use to boost just about anything, the evidence suggests that only a few ergogenic aids have consistently shown to be effective for improving athletic performance or altering body composition. These supplements include protein powders, creatine monohydrate, and buffering agents.

Protein powders

Protein powders are highly accessible and have been formulated to accommodate many dietary needs. Casein and whey are the two major proteins in cow's milk; the former constitutes 80 per cent of total protein in milk and the whey constitutes the remaining 20 per cent. Because whey is water-soluble and mixes easily, digestion occurs at a quicker rate, releasing amino acids into the bloodstream faster than casein, which is water insoluble. Casein also coagulates in the stomach and contains certain peptides that slow its digestion. Both milk-based proteins are well-documented and have been shown to be an effective strategy for increasing muscle mass and augmenting strength gains by increasing total daily protein intake when protein intake is suboptimal. Soy protein powder is another popular source of protein. Although soy has been shown to stimulate muscle protein synthesis better than casein, a 12-week resistance training and dietary supplementation study found that the milk-based proteins increased lean tissue and decreased fat tissue more than soy protein supplementation. However, nearly a decade later, a meta-analysis found no differences in strength gains or lean mass changes when comparing animal- and soy-based proteins. Other emerging plant-based protein sources include wheat, pea, and potato.

Creatine monohydrate

Creatine monohydrate is another popular and well-researched ergogenic aid that is widely accessible. Survey-based studies have reported that the prevalence of creatine use within athletic populations is about 15–40 per cent and more common in male strength-athletes. The role of creatine is to combine with phosphate to form phosphocreatine (PCr) and subsequently aid in the resynthesis of ATP for muscle contraction. Creatine can also enter the mitochondria, bind with ATP formed by the oxidative system, then re-enter the cytosol to buffer energy-needs. There are two main supplementation protocols for creatine monohydrate. The first requires creatine loading for 5–7 days (20g/day), followed by a maintenance dose of 3–5g/day. This will saturate creatine stores within the muscle and has been shown to increase high-intensity exercise, improve body composition and enhance recovery. The alternative strategy would be to ingest 3–5g/day for 28 days. Other notable clinical applications for creatine supplementation are being discovered and include recovery from certain injuries, brain and spinal cord neuroprotection, and maintaining heart function following ischemic heart disease.

Buffering agents

Buffering agents, such as bicarbonate and carnosine, have been shown to improve performance. Near maximal and maximal exercise increases the concentration of metabolic byproducts in the blood and muscle cells. This metabolic accumulation has been suggested to be one of many factors associated with fatigue. The body has its own buffering system; however, this system may be enhanced by supplemental sodium bicarbonate and beta-alanine. Firstly, sodium bicarbonate is a blood buffering agent that raises the pH (alkalizes the blood) helping hydrogen (H+) exit the muscle cell (buffering). Lowering H+ content within the muscle cells allows muscle contraction to continue. Sodium bicarbonate can be ingested a few hours before exercise at 0.3g/kg of bodyweight (22.5g for a 75kg dancer). Taste and side effects of this dosage should be considered. Carbon dioxide is produced with bicarbonate ingestion and can cause abdominal pain, flatulence, and diarrhoea. Therefore, supplementation can be taken with lower doses over a period of 3 days to 8 weeks. In contrast, beta-alanine is a precursor for carnosine synthesis and considered a powerful intracellular buffer regulating pH balance. Supplementation protocols for beta-alanine recommend 4–6g per day for a minimum of two weeks; 4 weeks have shown more benefits. Like creatine, this will saturate muscle tissue with carnosine. A very common side-effect of beta-alanine is paraesthesia, or a tingly feeling, shortly after consumption, lasting roughly 1 hour. Muscle buffering agents are mainly used to increase performance in sporting events that generally last 60–240 seconds.

REFERENCES

1. Kozai, A., Twitchett, E., Morgan, S., Wyon, M. (2020). 'Workload intensity and rest periods in professional ballet: Connotations for injury' in *International Journal of Sports Medicine* 41(6): 373–379. https//DOI:10.1055/a-1083-6539.
2. Howse, J. (1972). 'Orthopaedists Aid Ballet' in *Clinical Orthopaedics and Related Research* 89: 52–63.
3. Bowling, A. (1989). 'Injuries to dancers: Prevalence, treatment, and perceptions of causes' in *British Medical Journal (Clinical Research Edition)* 298: 731–734.
4. Brinson, P. and Dick, F. (1996). *Fit to Dance?* London: Calouste Gulbenkian Foundation.
5. Koutedakis, Y., Pacy, P.J., Carson, R.J., Dick, F. (1997). 'Health and fitness in professional dancers' in *Medical Problems of Performing Artists* 12(1): 23–27.
6. Koutedakis, Y., Khalouha, M., Pacy, P., Murphy, M., Dunbar, G. (1997). 'Thigh peak torques and lower-body injuries in dancers' in *Journal of Dance Medicine and Science* 1(1): 12–15.
7. Wyon, M., Abt, G., Redding, E., Head, A., Sharp, N. (2004). 'Oxygen uptake during modern dance class, rehearsal and performance' in *Journal of Strength and Conditioning Research* 18(3): 646–649. Doi:https://DOI:10.1519/13082.1
8. Laws, H. (2005). *Fit to Dance 2: Report of the Second National Inquiry into Dancers' Health and Injury in the UK*. London: Newgate Press.
9. Koutedakis, Y., Myszkewycz, L., Soulas, D., Papapostolou, V., Sullivan, I., Sharp, N.C. (1999). 'The effects of rest and subsequent training on selected physiological parameters in professional female classical dancers' in *International Journal of Sports Medicine* 20(6): 379–383. Doi:https://DOI:10.1055/s-2007-971148.
10. Twitchett, E., Angioi, M., Koutedakis, Y., Wyon, M. (2011). 'Do increases in selected fitness parameters affect the aesthetic aspects of classical ballet performance?' in *Medical Problems of Performing Artists* 26(1): 35–38.
11. Angioi, M., Metsios, G., Twitchett, E., Koutedakis, Y., Wyon, M. (2012). 'Effects of supplemental training on fitness and aesthetic competence parameters in contemporary dance: A randomised controlled trial' in *Medical Problems of Performing Artists* 27(1): 3–8.
12. Angioi, M., Metsios, G., Koutedakis, Y., Twitchett, E., Wyon, M. (2009). 'Physical fitness and severity of injuries in contemporary dance' in *Medical Problems of Performing Artists* 24(1): 26–29.
13. Twitchett, E., Brodrick, A., Nevill, A.M., Koutedakis, Y., Angioi, M., Wyon, M. (2010). 'Does physical fitness affect injury occurrence and time loss due to injury in elite vocational ballet students?' in *Journal of Dance Medicine and Science* 14(1): 26–31.
14. Nuttall, F.Q. (2015). 'Body mass index: Obesity, BMI, and health: A critical review' in *Nutrition Today* 50(3): 117–128.
15. Vuori, I. (1996). 'Peak bone mass and physical activity: A short review' in *Nutrition Reviews* 54(4): S11–S14.

REFERENCES

16. Amorim, T., Wyon, M., Maia, J., Machado, J., Marques, F., Metsios, G., Flouris, A., Koutedakis, Y. (2015). 'Prevalence of low bone mineral density in female dancers: A systematic review' in *Sports Medicine* 45(2): 257–268. Doi:10.1007/s40279-014-0268-5
17. Litonjua, A., Sparrow, D., Celedon, J., DeMolles, D., Weiss, S. (2002). 'Association of body mass index with the development of methacholine airway hyperresponsiveness in men: The Normative Aging Study' in *Thorax* 57(7): 581–585.
18. Bessonova, L., Marshall, S.F., Ziogas, A., Largent, J., Bernstein, L., Henderson, K.D., Ma, H., West, D.W., Anton-Culver, H. (2011). 'The association of body mass index with mortality in the California Teachers Study' in *International Journal of Cancer* 129(10): 2492–2501.
19. Twitchett, E., Angioi, M., Metsios, G., Koutedakis, Y., Wyon, M. (2008). 'Body composition and ballet injuries: A preliminary study' in *Medical Problems of Performing Artists* 23(3): 93–98.
20. Stokić, E., Srdić, B., Barak, O. (2005). 'Body mass index, body fat mass and the occurrence of amenorrhea in ballet dancers' in *Gynecological Endocrinology* 20(4): 195–199.
21. Amorim, T., Metsios, G.S., Flouris, A.D., Nevill, A., Gomes, T.N., Wyon, M., Marques, F., Nogueira, L., Adubeiro, N., Jamurtas, A.Z. (2019). 'Endocrine parameters in association with bone mineral accrual in young female vocational ballet dancers' in *Archives of Osteoporosis* 14(1): 46 Doi:https://doi.org/10.1007/s11657-019-0596-z
22. Komi, P., Viitasalo, J., Havu, M., Thorstensson, A., Sjödin, B., Karlsson, J. (1977). 'Skeletal muscle fibres and muscle enzyme activities in monozygous and dizygous twins of both sexes' in *Acta Physiologica Scandinavica* 100(4): 385–392.
23. Astrand, P., Rodahl, K. (1986). *Textbook of Work Physiology: Physiological Bases of Exercise*. 3rd ed. New York: McGraw-Hill International Editions.
24. Connolly, K., Forssberg, H. (1997). *Neurophysiology and Neuropsychology of Motor Development*. Cambridge: Mac Keith Press.
25. Schmidt, R., Wrisberg, C. (2000). *Motor Learning and Performance*. Champaign, Ill: Human Kinetics.
26. Lavoie, B., Devanne, H., Capaday, C. (1997). 'Differential control of reciprocal inhibition during walking versus postural and voluntary motor tasks in humans' in *Journal of Neurophysiology* 78(1): 429–438.
27. Dudley, D.A. (2015). 'A conceptual model of observed physical literacy' in *The Physical Educator* 72(5): 236–260.
28. Myer, G.D., Jayanthi, N., Difiori, J.P., Faigenbaum, A.D., Kiefer, A.W., Logerstedt, D., Micheli, L.J. (2015). 'Sport specialization, Part I: Does early sports specialization increase negative outcomes and reduce the opportunity for success in young athletes?' in *Sports Health* 7(5): 437–442.
29. Allen, N., Ribbans, W., Nevill, A.M., Wyon, M. (2014). 'Musculoskeletal injuries in dance: A systematic review' in *International Journal of Physical Medicine & Rehabilitation* 3(1): 1–8. Doi:http://dx.doi.org/10.4172/2329-9096.1000252
30. Wyon, M., Twitchett, E., Angioi, M., Clarke, F., Metsios, G., Koutedakis, Y. (2011). 'Time motion and video analysis of classical ballet and contemporary dance performance' in *International Journal of Sports Medicine* 32(11): 851–855. https//DOI:10.1055/s-0031-1279718.
31. Wyon, M. (2005). 'Cardiorespiratory training for dancers' in *Journal of Dance Medicine and Science* 9(1): 7–12.
32. Wyon, M., Koutedakis, Y. (2013). 'Muscular fatigue: Considerations for dancers' in *Journal of Dance Medicine and Science* 17(2): 77–83.
33. Koutedakis, Y. (2000). 'Burnout in dance: The physiological viewpoint' in *Journal of Dance Medicine and Science* 4(4): 122–127.
34. Selye, H. (1951). 'The general-adaptation-syndrome' in *Annual Review of Medicine* 2(1): 327–342.
35. Borg, G. (1978). 'Psychological assessments of physical effort' – paper presented at International Symposium on Psychological Assessment in Sport, Wingate Institute for Physical Education and Sport, Netanya, Israel.
36. Surgenor, B., Wyon, M. (2019). 'Measuring training load in dance: The construct validity of session-RPE' in *Medical Problems in Performing Artists* Doi:doi.org/10.21091/mppa.2019.1002
37. Apostolopoulos, N., Lahart, I., Plyley, M., Taunton, J., Nevill, A., Koutedakis, Y., Wyon,

REFERENCES

M., Metsios, G. (2018). 'The effects of different passive static stretching intensities on recovery from unaccustomed eccentric exercise: A randomized controlled trial' in *Applied Physiology, Nutrition, and Metabolism* https//DOI:10.1139/apnm-2017-0841

38. Tufano, J.J., Brown, L.E., Coburn, J.W., Tsang, K.K., Cazas, V.L., LaPorta, J.W. (2012). 'Effect of aerobic recovery intensity on delayed-onset muscle soreness and strength' in *The Journal of Strength & Conditioning Research* 26(10): 2777–2782.

39. Pearcey, G.E., Bradbury-Squires, D.J., Kawamoto, J.-E., Drinkwater, E.J., Behm, D.G., Button, D.C. (2015). 'Foam rolling for delayed-onset muscle soreness and recovery of dynamic performance measures' in *Journal of Athletic Training* 50(1): 5–13.

40. Best, T.M., Hunter, R., Wilcox, A., Haq, F. (2008). 'Effectiveness of sports massage for recovery of skeletal muscle from strenuous exercise' in *Clinical Journal of Sport Medicine* 18(5): 446–460.

41. Hohenauer, E., Taeymans, J., Baeyens, J.-P., Clarys, P., Clijsen, R. (2015). 'The effect of post-exercise cryotherapy on recovery characteristics: A systematic review and meta-analysis' in *PLOS One* 10(9): e0139028.

42. Wyon, M. (2014). 'Towards a new training methodology' in Brown, D., Vos, M. (eds): *Ballet, How and Why? On the Role of Classical Ballet in Dance Education*. Arnhem, Netherlands, ArtEZ Press: 111–118.

43. Croisier, J.-L. (2004). 'Muscular imbalance and acute lower extremity muscle injuries in sport' in *International SportMed Journal* 5(3): 169–176.

44. Cardinale, M., Newton, R., Nosaka, K. (2011). *Strength and Conditioning: Biological Principles and Practical Applications*. John Wiley & Sons.

45. Noakes, T.D. (2007). 'The central governor model of exercise regulation applied to the marathon' in *Sports Medicine* 37(4–5): 374–377.

46. Wyon, M., Redding, E., Abt, G., Head, A., Sharp, N.C.C. (2003). 'Development, reliability, and validity of a multistage dance specific aerobic fitness test (DAFT)' in *Journal of Dance Medicine and Science* 7(3): 80–84.

47. Twitchett, E., Nevill, A., Angioi, M., Koutedakis, Y., Wyon, M. (2011). 'The development of a multi-stage ballet-specific aerobic fitness test: Initial reliability and validity analysis' in *Journal of Dance Medicine and Science* 15(3): 123–127.

48. Apostolopoulos, N., Metsios, G., Flouris, A., Koutedakis, Y., Wyon, M. (2015). 'The relevance of stretch intensity and position: A systematic review' in *Frontiers in Psychology* 6:1128. https//DOI:10.3389/fpsyg.2015.01128.

49. Apostolopoulos, N., Metsios, G., Koutedakis, Y., Wyon, M. (2015). 'Stretch intensity vs. inflammation: A dose-dependent association?' in *International Journal of Kinesiology and Sports Science* 3(1): 1–5.

50. Boyle, M. (2016). *New Functional Training for Sports*. Human Kinetics.

51. Saeterbakken, A.H., Chaudhari, A., van den Tillaar, R., Andersen, V. (2019). 'The effects of performing integrated compared to isolated core exercises' in *PLOS One* 14(2): e0212216.

52. Butler, R.J., Hardy, L. (1992). 'The performance profile: Theory and application' in *The Sport Psychologist* 6: 253–264.

53. Redding, E., Wyon, M. (2007). *Dance Specific Fitness Tests*. London: Trinity Laban7.

54. McMillan, A., Proteau, L., Lèbe, R.-M. (1998). 'The effect of Pilates-based training on dancers' dynamic posture' in *Journal of Dance Medicine and Science* 2(3): 101–107.

55. Amorim, T.P., Sousa, F.M., dos Santos, J.A.R. (2011). 'Influence of Pilates training on muscular strength and flexibility in dancers' in *Motriz: Revista de Educação Física*. 17(4): 660–666.

56. Wang, Y.-T., Lin, P.-C., Huang, C.-F., Liang, L.-C., Lee, A.J. (2012). 'The effects of eight-week Pilates training on limits of stability and abdominal muscle strength in young dancers.' Paper presented at: Proceedings of World Academy of Science, Engineering and Technology.

57. Ahearn, E.L., Greene, A., Lasner, A. (2018). 'Some effects of supplemental Pilates training on the posture, strength, and flexibility of dancers 17 to 22 years of age' in *Journal of Dance Medicine and Science* 22(4): 192–202.

58. McLain, S., Carter C.L., Abel, J. (1997). 'The effect of a conditioning and alignment programme on the measurement of supine jump height and pelvic alignment when using the Current Concepts Reformer' in *Journal of Dance Medicine and Science* 1(4): 149–154.

173

INDEX

12-minute run test 52
5-10-5 agility test 52
Aerobic 31
   Foundation training 155
   Continuous training 32
   Cross-trainer 33
   Glycolysis 31, 33
   Running 33
   Oxidative pathway 32
Agility 20, 40, 43
All or Nothing Law 18
Amortization 41
Anaerobic 30
   Training 32, 33
   Buffering agents 170
   Carnosine 170
   High-intensity dance performance test 51
Artistic athletes 10
Back exercises
   Assisted chin ups 126
   Back extension 109, 110
   Bilateral bent-over row 135
   Bilateral pulldowns 137
   Bilateral seated row 135
   Chest supported incline dumbbell row 133
   Chin ups 127
   Kneeling single arm cable row 133
   Pull ups 128
   Rack pull 111
   Single arm dumbbell row 134
   Single arm lat pulldown 136
Balance 21
   Inverted y test 50
Body composition 13
   BMI 13
   Bone mineral density (BMD) 13
   Fat and health 14
Borg scale 23, 24
Box jumps 141
Bracing 44
Buffering agents 170

Burnout 28
Calf raise test 60
Calories 159
Carbohydrate 161
Cardiorespiratory training
   Aerobic training 32, 33
   Aerobic foundation training 155
   Anaerobic training 32, 33
   Borg scale 23, 24
   Circuit training 156
   Continuous training 32
   Cross-trainer 33
   Energy pathways 31
   Fitness 19, 29, 31
   Frequency 34
   Glycolysis 31, 33
   Oxidative pathway 32
   Progression 34
   Running 33
Carnosine 170
Causes of injury 11
Central adaptations 30
Chest supported incline dumbbell row 133
Chest Exercises
   Decline push up 123
   Dips 125
   Flat dumbbell press 129
   Incline dumbbell press 130
   Incline push up 121
   Push up 122
Chin ups 127
Circuit training 156
Closed kinetic chain movements 87
Concentric 18
Continuous training 32
Copenhagen side plank 81
Core
   Pelvic floor 44
Core training 43, 76
   Bear crawls 83
   Bird-dog 82
   Bird-dog with stability ball 83

Bracing 44
Back extension 109, 110
Copenhagen side plank 81
Dead bugs 76
Dead bugs with resistance 77
Forward ball rolls 78
Half kneeling Pallof press 84
Pike push ups 124
Plank 79
Reverse hyperextensions 107
Reverse plank 79
Shrimps 89
Side plank 80
Side plank with band 81
Standing Pallof press 85
Stir the pot 78
Suitcase carries 84
Creatine monohydrate 170
Cross-trainer 33
Dance Aerobic Fitness Test 34, 51
Dead bugs 76
Dead bugs with resistance 77
Decline push up 123
Delayed onset muscle soreness 27
Depth jumps 145
Depth jumps rebounds 143
Développé test 54
Diet induced thermogenesis 159
Digestion 158
Dips 125
Double leg stretch 74
Dynamic stretching 39
Early specialization 19
Eccentric contraction 18, 27
Elasticity 14
Endocrine 26, 28
Energy balance 159
Energy pathways 31
Ergogenic aids 169
   Creatine monohydrate 170

Bicarbonate 170
Essential amino acids 160
Essential fat 14
Exercise activity thermogenesis 159
Exercise order 65, 151
Extensibility 14
Exteroceptive feedback 17
Fast twitch fibre 16, 27
Fat 164
   Health 14
Fatigue 11, 31
   Fatigue resistance 36
Flat dumbbell press 129
Flexibility 21, 37
   Beighton test 53
   Développé test 54
   Dynamic stretching 39
   Golgi tendon organ (GTO) 17, 37
   Lying overhead reach test 56
   Modified Thomas Test 54
   Passive stretching 39
   Proprioceptive neuromuscular (PNF) stretching 40
Floor slide hamstring curls 117
Fluid intake 166
Foot contacts 42
Forward ball rolls 78
Foundation training 29
Free weights 35
Front foot elevated split squat 90
Front squat 100
Functional stability 21
General strength 34
Glute bridge 104
Glute ham raises 119
Glycogen 26
Glycolysis 31, 33
Goblet squat 98
Golgi tendon organ (GTO) 17, 37
Growth hormone (GH) 26

INDEX

Half kneeling Pallof press 84
Half roll down 71
Handstand push ups 124
Heart rate 23
   Training zones 32
High intensity intermittent training (HIIT) 30
   Aerobic 157
   Anaerobic 157
High-intensity dance performance test 51
Hip thrusts 105
Hundred 71
Hydration 46, 166
Hypertrophy 23
Incline dumbbell press 130
Incline push up 121
Individual differences 13, 14
Insulin-like growth factors (IGF) 26
Intermediate programmes 153
Inverted Y test 50
Iron 167
Isometric contraction 18
Jump rope 138
Ketogenic diet 165
Kinetic energy 41
Kneeling single arm cable row 133
Lateral lunge onto a step 95
Lateral split squats 92
Leg exercises
   Body weight squat 97
   Floor slide hamstring curls 117
   Front foot elevated split squat 90
   Front squat 100
   Glute bridge 104
   Glute ham raises 119
   Goblet squat 98
   Hip thrusts 105
   Lateral lunge onto a step 95
   Overhead squat 102
   Rear foot elevated split squats 93
   Reverse lunge off a step 95
   Single leg deadlift 106
   Single leg push jumps on low step 140
   Skater squat 88
   Stability ball hamstring curl 115
   Staggered stance deadlift 113
   Step ups 87
   Sumo deadlift 114
   Trap bar deadlift 112
   Trap-bar squat 99
   Walking lunges 96

Lunge onto a step 94
Lying overhead reach test 56
Maintenance training 25
Maximum strength 34
Medicine ball
   Backwards throws 149
   Lateral slams 147
   Oblique toss 147
   Slams 147
   Test 57
   Throw 146
Micronutrients 167
Modified thomas test 54
Motor learning 17
Movement
   Closed kinetic chain 87
   Concentric 18
   Control 17
   Speed 42
Muscle 14
   Agonist 18
   Anatomy 15
   Antagonist 18
   Assistant agonist 18
   Concentric contraction 18
   Eccentric contraction 18, 27
   Elasticity 14
   Endurance 19, 35, 36
   Extensibility 14
   Fast twitch fibre 16, 27
   Fatigue resistance 36
   Fibres 16
   Glycogen 26, 162, 168
   Golgi Tendon Organ (GTO) 17, 37
   Hypertrophy 23
   Irritability 15
   Isometric contraction 18
   Kinetic energy 41
   Motor learning 17
   Movement control 17
   Muscle spindles 17, 37
   Neutralizer 18, 29
   Organization 13, 16
   Parallel elastic component (PEC) 14
   Peripheral adaptations 30
   Power 19, 30, 35
   Properties 14
   Proprioceptive feedback 17
   Series elastic component (SEC) 14, 30
   Slow twitch fibre 16, 27, 36
   Stabilizer 18, 29
   Strength 19, 29
   Structure 13
   Tension 15
Needs analysis 19

Fit to Dance survey 12
Performance profiling 47
Neuromuscular 20, 23, 27, 30
   All or Nothing law 18
   Amortization 41
   Movement control 17
Neutralizer muscle 18, 29
Non-exercise activity thermogenesis 159
Nutrition 46, 158
   Muscle glycogen 162, 168
   Buffering agents 170
   Calories 159
   Carbohydrate 161
   Carnosine 170
   Creatine monohydrate 170
   Diet induced thermogenesis 159
   Digestion 158
   Energy balance 159
   Ergogenic aids 169
   Essential amino acids 160
   Essential fat 14
   Exercise activity thermogenesis 159
   Fat 164
   Fluid intake 166
   Hydration 46, 166
   Iron 167
   Ketogenic diet 165
   Micronutrients 167
   Non-exercise activity thermogenesis 159
   Pre-performance carbohydrate 163
   Protein 160
   Protein powder 169
   Relative energy deficit in sport (RED-S) 158, 168
   Resting metabolic rate 159
   Storage fat 14
   Vitamin D 167
One leg circle 72
Overhead squat 102
Overhead squat test 62
Overtraining 12, 27
Oxidative pathway 32
Parallel elastic component (PEC) 14
Passive stretching 39
Pelvic floor 44
Performance enhancement 11, 31
Performance profiling 47
Peripheral adaptations 30
Physical literacy 19, 22
Pike push ups 124

Pilates 44
Pilates exercises
   Double leg stretch 74
   Half roll down 71
   Hundred 71
   Mat work 68
   One leg circle 72
   Reformer 68
   Roll up 72
   Rolling like a ball 72
   Single leg stretch 73
   Spine stretch forward 75
Pilates history 67
Pilates principles 68, 69
   Breath 69
   Centring 69
   Concentration 69
   Control 69
   Flow 69
   Precision 69
Plank 79
Plank test 58
Plyometrics 40, 138
   Foot contacts 42
   Kinetic energy 41
Plyometric exercises
   Box jumps 141
   Depth jumps 145
   Depth jumps rebounds 143
   Jump rope 138
   Medicine ball backwards throws 149
   Medicine ball oblique toss 147
   Medicine ball lateral slams 147
   Medicine ball slams 147
   Pogo hops 139
   Push ups 145
   Reverse drop jumps off a low step 139
   Skater jumps 140
   Skipping 138
   Squat jumps 143
Pogo hops 139
Power naps 146
Power
   Muscle 19, 30, 35
   Training 36
Pre-performance carbohydrate 163
Press up test 59
Proprioceptive neuromuscular stretching (PNF) 40
Programmes
   Advanced 154
   Agility training 43
   Beginner 152
   Body weight training 35
   Borg Scale 23, 24

INDEX

Cardiorespiratory training frequency 34
Cardiorespiratory training progression 34
Central adaptations 30
Circuit training 156
Continuous training 32
Design 64, 150
Exercise order 65, 151
Heart rate zones 32
High intensity intermittent training (HIIT) 30
HIIT aerobic 157
HIIT anaerobic 157
Intermediate 153
Rate of perceived exertion (RPE) 23, 24, 32
Reps in reserve 151
Sets 151
Tempo 152
Protein 160
Protein powder 169
Pull up test 60
Pull ups 128
Push up 122
Quality, not quantity 64
Rack pull 111
Range of movement (ROM) 37
Rate of perceived exertion (RPE) 23, 24, 32
Rear foot elevated split squats 93
Recovery 25, 26, 27
  Delayed onset muscle soreness (DOMS) 27
  Endocrine 26, 28
  Growth hormone (GH) 26
  Insulin-like growth factors (IGF) 26
  Power naps 46
  Sleep 28
  Swimming 33
  Testosterone 26
Reformer 68
Relative energy deficit in sport (RED-S) 158, 168
Relative strength 34
Repetitions 36, 151
Reps in reserve 151
Resistance bands 35
Rest 21, 23, 27, 151
  Power naps 46
  Sleep 28
Resting metabolic rate 159

Reverse drop jumps off a low step 139
Reverse hyperextensions 107
Reverse lunge off a step 95
Reverse plank 79
Roll up 72
Rolling like a ball 72
Romberg test 79
Running 33
Schedules 28
Screening 29
Seated overhead press 131
Series elastic component (SEC) 14, 30
Sets 151
Shoulder
  Internal external rotation test 56
  Handstand push ups 124
  Seated overhead press 131
  Standing overhead press 131
Shrimps 89
Side plank 80
Side plank with band 81
Single arm dumbbell row 134
Single arm lat pulldown 136
Single leg deadlift 106
Single leg push jumps on low step 140
Single leg stretch 73
Sit-up test 59
Skater jumps 140
Skater squat 88
Skipping 138
Sleep 28
Slow twitch fibre 16, 27, 36
Specific strength 35
Spine stretch forward 75
Split squat 90
Squat jumps 143
Stability 21
Stability ball hamstring curl 15
Stabilizer 18, 29
Staggered stance deadlift 113
Standing overhead press 131
Standing Pallof press 85
Star excursion test 50
Step ups 87
Stir the pot 78
Storage fat 14
Strength 19, 29
Stretch 26, 37
  Duration 38
  Intensity 38

Lengthening reaction 37
  Order 38
  Position 38
  Reflex 37
Stretching exercises
  Active 39
  Aggressive 40
  Ballistic 40
  Passive 39
  Proprioceptive neuromuscular (PNF) 40
Suitcase carries 84
Sumo deadlift 114
Supercompensation 27
Supplemental training 28
Swimming 33
Tempo 152
Tendons 14
Tension 15
Tests 29, 47
  12-minute run 52
  5-10-5 agility 52
  Back extension test 59
  Beighton test 53
  Calf raise test 60
  Dance aerobic fitness test 34, 51
  Flexibility developpe test 54
  High-intensity dance performance 51
  Inverted Y 50
  Lying overhead reach 56
  Maximum strength 34
  Medicine ball 57
  Modified Thomas 54
  Overhead squat 62
  Performance profiling 47
  Plank 58
  Press up 59
  Pull up 60
  Range of movement (ROM) 37
  Romberg 49
  Shoulder internal external rotation 56
  Sit-up 59
  Star excursion 50
  Triple hop 61
  Vertical jump 57
Testosterone 26
Time under tension 23
Training age 11, 22
Training impulse (TRIMPS) 23, 24
Training phases 29
Training stimulus 22
Training
  Age 11, 22

Central adaptations 30
Energy pathways 31
Exercise order 65, 151
Fatigue resistance 36
Flexibility 21, 37
Foundation 29
Free weights 35
Fun 66
Functional stability 21
General strength 34
Heart rate 23
Heart rate zones 32
Individual differences 13, 14
Isometric 35
Maintenance 25
Maximum strength 34
Medicine ball 45
Movement speed 42
Muscle endurance 35, 36
Overtraining 12, 27
Performance enhancement 11, 31
Peripheral adaptations 30
Phases 29
Physical literacy 19, 22
Plyometrics 40, 138
Power 36
Quality, not quantity 64
Rate of perceived exertion (RPE) 23, 24, 32
Relative strength 34
Repetitions 36, 151
Schedules 28
Specific strength 35
Supercompensation 27
Supplemental 28
Tempo 152
Time under tension 23
Training impulse (TRIMPS) 23, 24
Warm-down 26
Weight moved 23, 37
Weighted training 35
Weights machines 35
Work:rest ratio 23, 32
Trap bar deadlift 112
Trap-bar squat 99
Triple hop test 61
Vertical jump 57
Vitamin D 167
Walking lunges 96
Warm-down 26
Weight moved 23, 37
Weighted training 35
Weights machines 35
Work:rest ratio 23, 32